Dr Herbert Dardik's endorsement:

This is the book that I would have wanted to have written. Plain homespun philosophy mixed with seasoned experience is at the core of this book, providing a practical no-nonsense approach when it comes to choosing a doctor and then staying on top of the situation. Dr. George LeMaitre clearly belongs to the genre of doctors who base care on humanistic values, relationships and common sense. It is refreshing to revisit the doctor-patient relationship in light of our current schism between provider and consumer, which appears to forever widen with the help of the third-party payers. Paradigm shifts in all of medicine tend to focus on high-tech impersonal care. Optimal care will only come about if we additionally heed the words of Dr. George LeMaitre. I would mandate this book as required reading for all our politicians and legislators.

Dr. Dardik's credentials:

Professor of Surgery
Mount Sinai Hospital and Medical Center
University of Pennsylvania

Chief, Departments of Surgery and Vascular Surgery
Englewood Hospital and Medical Center
Englewood, New Jersey

CHOOSING YOUR DOCTOR

TWENTY CRITICAL CHECK POINTS

George D. LeMaitre, M.D., F.A.C.S.

ISBN 0-7414-4552-2

Book cover design by Suki Soltysik, based on illustration by Christopher Fotino

Published by:

INFINITY
PUBLISHING.COM

1094 New DeHaven Street, Suite 100
West Conshohocken, PA 19428-2713
Info@buybooksontheweb.com
www.buybooksontheweb.com
Toll-free (877) BUY BOOK
Local Phone (610) 941-9999
Fax (610) 941-9959

Printed in the United States of America

Printed on Recycled Paper

Published December 2008

To an unforgettable friend and colleague

...my Dad...!

Table of Contents

Stop!

new

Check your ^ doctor carefully—Very Carefully!

Read this book like a road map, something you store in the glove compartment of your car and refer to it often whenever you visit your doctor. Read a chapter here and there, think about its message, and apply it to your new doctor every time you see him or her.

Heath insurance systems are managing your doctor intensively, almost demanding that he ration your health care to save money. They want the doctor to limit the number of referrals, limit the number of tests and, especially, the number of hospitalizations carried out on your behalf.

To paraphrase an old saying, they are saying to your doctor: "Don't just do something Doctor, stand there".

I call these insurance systems the new HMOs: "Handcuffed Medical Organizations" for that is what they are trying to do to your doctor.

The whole point of this book is to teach you how you can manage your doctor and beat the insurance system. I want you to tell your doctor, in so many unspoken words, how he or she is to: "Do something, doctor, don't just stand there."

If you learn nothing else from this book, learn that the key to managing your doctor is to carry a small notebook and pen with each visit to your doctor. Open it up and write down things he is telling you. This will send a powerful message that you take these visits and his words very seriously.

Prologue

At 2:47 a.m., Tuesday, July 2, exactly 3 hours and 17 minutes after he was admitted to Memorial Hospital's emergency room, Henry J., 45 year-old father of four children, was pronounced dead. The coroner would ascribe his death to "acute respiratory arrest secondary to subdural hematoma" (hemorrhage in the brain), but the physicians who labored those three hours to save Henry would find that his death was totally unnecessary—the fatal outcome had been set in motion three months earlier; one of their colleagues, Dr. M., was at least partially to blame. **Mr. J.'s widow would never find out what happened.**

HENRY'S STORY...

Henry was brought to the emergency room by ambulance at 11:30, Monday evening. He was in a coma.

"He has been acting strangely all day," his wife told the emergency-room physician. "He said he had a bad headache; he felt dizzy, couldn't keep his balance."

The physician noticed large bruises all over Henry's body. Mrs. J., who had noticed the marks three days earlier, had called her physician. "He couldn't tell what they were over the phone," she said. "So he gave Henry an appointment for next week."

"About three months ago," Mrs. J. explained, "Henry dropped a heavy crate on his leg. Over the next three days the entire leg became swollen. I took him to the emergency room and they told me he had a blood clot; phlebitis they called it.

Our physician was on vacation so the HMO referred us to a surgeon on their roster. He prescribed something to thin Henry's blood. I asked whether Henry should be in the hospital but the surgeon said it wasn't necessary. I don't remember the name of the medicine; it was a little round, white pill. He told Henry to take one a day and get his blood checked weekly. He examined my husband every two weeks to be sure his blood was thin enough. The swelling in Henry's leg went down and he has been well... until tonight"

Mrs. J. had no idea what caused the bruises all over her husband's body. He had been complaining of arthritis for a week," she said, "and was taking a lot of aspirin."

"Aspirin?" The emergency room physician was excited. "How much aspirin? How much did he take?"

"Oh, a lot—maybe eight a day. He said they weren't working. He joked about wholesale aspirin not being worth much."

"Did the surgeon tell you anything about the blood thinner?" he asked. "What was the name of the drug?"

"No, he said it would help cure the phlebitis. He said Henry would have to get a blood test every week to see how thin his blood was."

"Was the drug called Coumeral?"

"Yes, That was it—Coumeral! I remember now."

"Did the surgeon tell you anything about the hazards of Coumeral?"

"No," she said, "only that Henry had to remember to take it each day."

"Did he tell you or Henry not to take any other pills, such as aspirin, while on Coumeral?"

"No. He told us nothing else."

WHAT KILLED HENRY?

The emergency room physician now had his lead. There were black and blue spots all over Henry J.'s body. A blood test showed that his blood was too thin. The diagnosis was also too clear. Henry J. had bled into his brain from an overdose of Coumeral. He had also bled under his skin, hence the appearance of bruises.

But the overdose of Coumeral, how come? Surely Mrs. J. had seen to it that her husband had taken one pill a day, the prescribed amount. And the weekly blood test—the surgeon had told Mrs. J repeatedly that his blood was precisely as thin as he wanted it, and that he should continue to take one Coumeral a day.

The villain was aspirin. Aspirin is incompatible with Coumeral because it increases the blood-thinning effects of the drug. Henry J. had been taking aspirin for almost one week prior to his death. **The aspirin along with the Coumeral had proven lethal**.

Why hadn't the surgeon told Mr. and Mrs. J. to avoid all pills incompatible with Coumeral, particularly aspirin, such a commonly used pill?

Why wasn't Mr. J.'s primary care physician more curious about the black and blue marks when Mrs. J. called and described them on the phone? Why didn't he know his patient was on Coumeral? Shouldn't he have asked more questions over the phone? Should he have seen Mr. J. sooner?

Why hadn't the emergency room surgeon notified Mr. J.'s family doctor that he had placed his patient on Coumeral?

Should the emergency-room staff have notified Mr. J.'s doctor after he returned from vacation that they had referred his patient to a surgeon on the emergency call roster?

What went wrong? Who was to blame for this tragedy? What is wrong with the communication system among some doctors that allows this misinformation to occur? What could have been done differently? **What can YOU do to prevent this tragedy from happening to your loved one or yourself?**

These are the questions that led me to write this book.

Introduction

Many people choose a doctor with little more thought than they give to selecting a brand of aspirin. Some run their fingers through the yellow pages and stop at a name that appeals to them. Others get their advice from neighbors, coworkers or their hair stylists. One of my patients chose me because he had seen me on television and liked the way I spoke.

Such casual approaches aren't unusual. Many people feel the choice isn't that important, that all doctors are equal and the choice is only a matter of personal taste, convenience or price. Most Americans have an abiding faith in the designation "M.D." As long as it comes after a person's name, he or she is a certified healer.

Where do people get the idea that all doctors are equal? I don't know the origin of this belief, but it certainly has been perpetuated by the long-standing ethical premise that forbids doctors to criticize their colleagues. **There is almost a total conspiracy of silence about the incompetent physician.** Criticism of professional failure has not been a policy of the American Medical Association or the medical schools, and I believe this is an abdication of their responsibility to the public. **You cannot imagine the criticism I received from Medical societies with the first edition of this book.**

Why don't people put the same effort into choosing a physician as they do in choosing a new car? They shop around, compare models and costs and choose the one that suits them best. As consumers, people today are increasingly sophisticated and informed, except when it comes to choosing a doctor.

Should you worry about your choice of doctor? Yes, you're damned right you should. The bald fact is that your choice can mean the difference between life or death for you or some member of your family. If you had your choice between a bad doctor or no doctor at all, you'd be better off taking care of yourself. A bad doctor can be a disaster in your life.

Should you be concerned about HMOs and how your company contracts with them and limits your choice of doctors? Of course you should! What is this thing called CAPITATION MEDICINE and how does it affect your medical care, for better or for worse?

How do doctors differ? What makes one good and another bad? Eighty years ago the answer was simple: Good doctors graduated from good medical schools, bad ones "graduated" from diploma mills, where they bought their degrees. Today, thanks to a revolution in medical education, there are no more diploma mills. All medical schools are good, and almost all doctors have good credentials. The differences between good and bad ones are more subtle, more personal, harder to detect but just as critical for you.

The yellow pages are a place to start your search but won't tell you which doctors are good and which are bad. Your neighbors, coworkers and hair stylists aren't going to know either. **To choose a good doctor, you need to know what to look for, what's important, and what you can ignore. That's where this book can help.**

And don't be fooled by employers who say you have no choice; that the HMO determines whom you will see. I call HMOs "Handcuffed Medical Organizations." Read on and you will find out more and how to undo the handcuffs.

Preface to Second Edition

To say that things have changed significantly in the twenty years since I first wrote this book would be to state the ludicrously obvious. The changes make any recasting of my book seemingly impossible and suggest the need for an entirely different book.

I do not think this is the case on closer examination. Indeed, before I speak of changes I should clear up a misconception many readers had from the first edition. Somehow they came to believe the doctor I described as the 'good doctor' truly existed and it was a matter of fingerprinting my book version and looking for the real one out there.

The doctor I described in 1979 never existed. He was an ideal, a construct of my mind, something one sought as medical perfection but could never find. Let me say where that ideal physician came from and then we can go on to the changes that have occurred in these past 20 years.

I will begin with my dad, a general practitioner in a small community from 1929 until 1969. His office was in our home, three out of ten rooms serving as his waiting room, his consulting room and his examining room. He saw patients in those rooms four weekdays each week from 2-4 pm and 7-9 pm. We often heard him from our kitchen.

His day began early, around 7; he made two to three hours of house calls, a two-hour visit to the small hospital where he had operating room privileges, and then his office. He went back on house calls after 4 p.m. His day was long. He had no associates to cover his practice, no answering service to screen his calls, no pagers, no cellular phones.

He had no secretaries, no nurses, no bookkeepers. He did all this alone, examined patients without chaperones, had no malpractice insurance and was not sued in forty years of active practice. His family life suffered; ask me!

His payments were often in barter—baskets of food and fruit, free car service, free movies, even free restaurant meals

The house call served as the focal point of his practice, the place where he came to know the most about his patients. I distinctly recall his asking me (maybe at age 9) to look in the medicine cabinet at a patient's home. There were dozens upon dozens of half-empty, filthy, unlabelled medicine bottles. He asked me to check the refrigerator; the food had an odor and the refrigerator ice box was in horrendous condition. These were largely poor, immigrant patients without an education. He learned of their health needs by these *home visits*, as he preferred to call them. **The dangerous medicine cabinet and the malodorous icebox told him more about the health hazards facing his patients than the stethoscope and the thermometer.**

Was my dad different from most docs of his day? Of course not; there were many, many like him. Their scientific knowledge was feeble compared to doctors of the post-war years. Their knowledge of patients was masterful. **They were long on heart and short on science**, and I do not mean this in any derogatory sense.

When I entered my practice my dad and his colleagues were slowly hanging up their shingles. I worked with some of them, learned their ways, extracted what I could from their long suits, and avoided their short suits. Several acted as my mentors and, by 1975, seeing some of their weaknesses and the failings of modern medicine, I embarked on the first edition of my book. I spanned medicine from 1900 through 1975, choosing what I saw to be the good, leaving aside the bad.

The good doctor was, therefore, an ideal, not a real doctor. I saw efforts made in the '70s and '80s to eliminate the bad things in medicine, especially the rising cost of health care caused by a great deal of unnecessary medicine and surgery practiced then.

In the '90's I saw the opposite image, as cost-cutters had taken over the practice of medicine and brought about the demise of necessary medicine and surgery. **Choice of doctors began to suffer**.

The whole thing might seem impossible to sort out; much of the obfuscation in the media is unnecessary. Simple issues are made complex, often by people with hidden agendas.

I am going to attempt to clarify this by taking each chapter of my 1979 book, emphasizing the points that still remain valid, but pointing out some of the faults that have developed in the system **and how you, the patient, can get to manage these problems**. A great tragedy is unfolding and needs a very serious overview by the public, not trusting the politicians, the insurance industry or organized Medicine.

Plan for This Second Edition

I will take each chapter of my 1979 *Good Doctor* book, add some necessary changes, and then do a **time out** where I will try to show, as simply as I can, what has been happening to the practice of Medicine.

These "time outs" are meant to give you a chance to see some of the contradictions that may exist even in some of the concepts I am promulgating here. That is how fast things change, and it is arrogance for any writer about medicine to assume he or she knows the future.

Here I hope to act for the reader and evaluate again what I said twenty years before and am saying now. I plan to update you about how things stand but I am also suggesting that you should take some of what seemed valid to me twenty years earlier with a large grain of salt. I am hoping, with the advantage of a retrospective gaze, to make a serious point about the gravity of the current situation and how it has often destroyed any meaningful definition of the good doctor or the chance to arrive at that free choice I advocated two decades earlier or even now. I am also hoping that these time-outs imply a less than dogmatic point of view, as times, medical economics and medical legislation go on at lightning speed around us. **In short, none of what I say is written in stone and all will change almost as I write.** I am also suggesting that you put on your thinking cap and pretend you are engaged with me in a dialogue.

I will intentionally repeat myself throughout this book and will not listen to my editors who dislike repetition. **The only way to really get things across in such short books is to repeat and repeat**.

I hope my simple goal, to clarify the issue and lay it before the public, will be accomplished. What you do about it is up to you. There will be trade offs and you will have to decide which way you wish our profession to go.

Chapter 1: The Evolution of Health Care

"you must remember this..."

Chapter summary: My father was an old-time general practitioner—a family doctor—and I sometimes made house calls with him when I was growing up. As a child I was surrounded by his colleagues and heard their war stories. Later, in medical school, I learned their strengths and weaknesses. The GP knew his patients as people and as families but he lacked a thorough knowledge of scientific medicine.

After the Second World War, the specialist displaced the generalist. They knew more about particular areas of the human body but less about the patient and family. In the 1980s *managed care* promised to resurrect the primary care physician who would know all about his or her patients and control cost by eliminating useless and overspecialized medical care.

Tragically, today, cost cutters and number crunchers are running the show and they care more about profits than patients. So we are back to square one: the primary care physician alone, isolated, and unable to make proper use of specialists.

Why We Loved the Old GP

There was something about the "old time doc" of happy memory that people seem to miss. Older patients remember a far more humane, personable, and less mercenary doctor who seems to have answered most of their needs, made house calls and served as their counselor. He has become a misty legend among younger people who believe that the old doctor was far superior to the modern doctor.

This physician cared for his patients in a very personal way and offered them a sense of permanence, **a continuity of care**. He seemed comfortable treating the majority of illnesses. When a specialist was needed, he considered himself responsible for seeking him out, while remaining the anchorman. There is security in knowing that your medical team has a captain or a manager, the job the primary physician did so well. He acted as a go-between, a contact man between the patient and the specialist. He put in plain English what the specialist was saying and reduced the whole arrangement to a workable, human, and intensely personal operation. In effect, he created a rational system for his patients without depersonalizing medical care. He was called a general practitioner or, in modern jargon, a primary care physician.

Fast Forward to the great specialist glut: 1950s and 60s

By the late 1950s we had all but eliminated the primary-care physician. We assumed that all medicine needed was a series of high-powered specialists to cover each area of the human body, one piece at a time. The result was a hodgepodge of ever-multiplying and specialized physicians who, individually, refused to consider the whole patient their responsibility.

Someone worked on John Smith's middle ear and someone checked his diabetes; someone worried about his marital troubles and someone else his gallbladder. But no one considered John Smith. **Specialists might diagnose *disease* but it takes a committed primary care physician, interested in the patient and his entire family, to manage *dis-ease*.** We had thrown the baby out with the bathwater.

No matter how hard we tried to tell people they were better off with a string of specialists, they pushed for a primary or personal physician. This was not a longing for the past. It was a sustained demand for something we had eliminated, something we didn't allow for in our plans for the utopian health delivery system. **People were looking for a human being who cared about them, not some starry-eyed professor, meandering about in a long white lab coat**, who dogmatically fitted them into a specialty slot and told them to move this way or that. They wanted an anchorman who could put together the whole thing called health maintenance.

The number of super-specialists continued to multiply like rabbits. This produced a health delivery system best described as a mess. Patients were left with no one physician to whom they could turn and hold accountable for their total care. This led to confusion, duplication of expensive and sometimes dangerous services, conflicts in the use of drugs, buck-passing, depersonalization. The problem of overspecialization ran very deep and negated the very concept of a sacred doctor-patient relationship upon which the whole tradition of the physician rests. The psychological makeup of the specialist who fancied himself or herself an expert in one area of the body prevented the development of the personal approach that excellent medical care demands. The old family doctor knew instinctively that there was a mystical but real relationship between a person's illness and his or her lifestyle. He knew that family quarrels, work tensions and the strains of living affected his patient's physical and mental health, and he kept this in mind as he treated the illness at hand. **He knew these things because he was a doctor, friend and confidant for all his patients.** His house calls were more than a convenience. They helped him size up the entire life-space situation of his patients in ways totally unavailable to the impersonal, nine-to-five, aloof super-specialist of today.

The GP knew too little about too much

I thought and wrote despairingly of the demise of the family doctor in the late '70s but I was not advocating a return to the past. The old general practitioner, including my dad, could not be resurrected. The knowledge explosion made it impossible for one doctor to take care of his patients from cradle to grave—from obstetrics through pediatrics to major medical and surgical illnesses. **Specialization was a consequence of the rapidly expanding body of medical knowledge.** Efforts to reverse the trend would have been anti-scientific and would have negated the progress in medical science that was extending our lives and making many diseases tolerable, if not curable. **The best doctor for a serious middle-ear disease was, and is, a middle-ear specialist.**

The specialist knew too much about too little

Still, there were certain basic truths about medical care that we lost. The specialist view is necessarily narrow. He has a sustained interest in his narrow field of expertise but does not feel responsible for areas outside his professional domain. Specialists pass the patient, bucket-brigade fashion, from one to another, none feeling responsible for managing the whole team.

A primary-care physician, on the contrary, remains responsible for your care regardless of how many specialists are called in. You depend on her for guidance through the increasingly complex medical delivery system existing today. She made certain that specialists were not issuing conflicting orders, incompatible drugs and confusing recommendations. **I like to think of a primary-care physician as a team manager or orchestra conductor, since this implies that she occupies the foremost spot in the medical team that takes care of you and keeps the whole team together … the orchestra in tune.**

My house call experiences with dad

I made house calls with my dad when I was nine to twelve years old. I vividly recall his telling me there was a difference between the house call and the home visit: **"The house call is why they asked you to come, son. The home visit is why you should be there!"** He meant, as I later understood, that he made a house call to serve the immediate need of the patient. But he looked upon it as a home visit, a time to assess the overall health practices of the family and a time to bond on a far deeper level than his office could engender. I knew none of these distinctions then, of course. I learned the value of the home visits long after they became an anachronism. Physicians do not make house calls any more. The visits were inefficient and not very scientific. There is very little medical science that a doctor can possibly carry in his black bag. Alas, the home visit died with the house call, and this was a real tragedy.

The home visit helped reduce the professional barriers that separate a doctor from his patients. The physician became a friend of each of his patients and not separated from them by the pomp and circumstance of his profession and the artificial barriers induced by the sterile atmosphere of his office. There is no doubt in my mind that the home visit served this purpose quite well, a valid aspect that has been lost.

I can't say I enjoyed the house calls because they often came when I would have preferred a baseball game. Dad dragged me along to keep him company. Now I'm glad I made those trips. I have such pleasant memories and I learned a lot about the warm connection he had with his patients, connections that could only come about by making house calls. Frequently I would go into the house and stay in the kitchen while my dad went into the sick room to examine his patient. The spouse would often give me a piece of cake or pie and I would sit there, feeling a bit strange, talking with members of the family until my dad reappeared. He would often sit down at the kitchen table and have pie and coffee with the family. The conversation was more often about politics (my father's favorite topic) than about the illness he was treating. I sensed an equality between him and his patients who, when they disagreed with his political views, often argued with him at the kitchen table. You see, he was on equal ground, visiting "on their turf" so to speak. This could never happen in his office where, propped up behind a mahogany desk and surrounded by the sights and sounds of Medicine, patients would not dare talk with him about these subjects.

More about the docs of old

Let's look at history. If you were to open a 1940 telephone book and check the yellow pages, you would have to search hard to find a doctor who specialized in anything. Almost all of them were general practitioners or what we now call family doctors. You simply read: Robert Smith, MD and then followed something about his office hours, address, and telephone number. These doctors delivered babies and took care of young children, adults, and the elderly. They did surgery, examined your eyes, nose, and throat and so forth; they held office hours for any and all comers and made house calls and nursing home visits. They covered the emergency rooms, which were staffed by nurses who called the doctors at home when an emergency came in. Most community hospitals had no full-time emergency room doctors.

It doesn't take a rocket scientist to realize that, by the specialty standards that were to evolve shortly after the Second World War, these family doctors may have known their patients extremely well but their knowledge of the science of medicine was certainly paltry. Modern medical science is just too complex for one doctor to know it all.

The rise of specialism

Now check the yellow pages, say around 1950. Specialties are beginning to appear after the name of the doctor. The five major specialties to enter the 1950 scene were obstetrics/ gynecology, internal medicine, general surgery, and pediatrics, along with the eye, ear, nose, and throat specialists. The general practitioner or family doctor existed in great numbers but folks were choosing specialists more and more for their care.

The hospitals responded by severely limiting what the general practitioner could do. Gone were the days when he could do major surgery one day, deliver babies the next, care for young babies and children, and care for extensive geriatric medical problems. My dad related a heart-rending, somewhat sardonic story that illustrates this change. He was about to deliver a woman in active labor and, at the last minute, realized that forceps would be necessary for what was turning into a more complex delivery than he had foreseen. Unbeknownst to him, after he asked the circulating nurse for the forceps, she had notified her supervisor who called the Chief of Obstetrics. Rules had changed. My dad did not realize that now only certified obstetricians were allowed to place forceps on the patient. The obstetrician appeared in the operating room and informed my dad that he was not allowed to insert the forceps. Shocked at this new twist in his life, my dad looked angrily at the obstetrician and stated, as he left the room in a furious rage, **"John, I delivered you 39 years ago."**

Prices rose dramatically to pay for all this specialized care but the government or the insurance companies were almost totally footing the bill and so no one seemed to care what it all cost. **"Spare no expense, doctor, I want the best"** was a frequent nostrum. If not spoken openly, it certainly was on every patient's mind.

Time Out!

The Second World War movie *Casablanca* features a beautiful, romantic song called *As Time Goes By.* The words remain imprinted in my memory as the lead actress sings unforgettable lyrics such as **"You must remember this, a kiss is still a kiss, a sigh is still a sigh..."**

In spite of the great roles played by Humphrey Bogart and Ingrid Bergman, things do change and nothing remains the same *as time goes by*. Medicine continues to evolve. When I wrote of primary-care physicians in1979, I pointed out that the trend was towards too much specialization. I had hoped that, with the advent of so-called managed care, the role of the primary-care physician would be enhanced and we would see a proper proportion of specialty care return, something that surely existed in the first 50 or 60 years of the 20th century.

Alas, it did not work out that way. When I also pointed out that the best doctor for a serious middle-ear infection was a middle-ear specialist I sensed that once the number crunchers got control of medical care the less expensive primary care doc would be called upon to do things he or she was simply not equipped by training or experience to do, take care of serious, middle-ear infection, and so forth.

Over the course of the next three decades, from 1950 to1980, the move toward specialized care became greatly overdone, something I also hastened to mention in the first edition of this book. It started to become absurd how many specialists a patient would see in the course of an illness. None of these specialists had a good idea of the patient's health status, each concentrated instead on his or her specialized area of the body. The joke around town, often containing a grain of truth, was that you needed a doctor who specialized in left leg pain for a pain in your left leg and a doctor who specialized in right arm pain for a pain in your right arm.

In 1979 we were in the throes of converting from a system of unmanaged to one of managed care. It was my hope, although I was very skeptical, that the cost overruns of overspecialized care would finally lead to a rational system of managed care, in which physicians, insurance companies and government would work out a proper balance between primary medical care and specialized care. I had hoped that the over-emphasis in specialized care would yield to a proper balance between the wisdom and experience of the primary-care physician and the intensive expertise of his or her specialized counterpart. I hoped that a careful working together would give us the best of all worlds.

Alas, the situation has grown from bad to worse over these last three decades. Indeed, managed care, as constructed by industry and health insurance companies, heavily marketed the idea that the primary-care physician was best prepared to care for the majority of patients' problems and that the specialist should be brought in only when necessary. I felt this position was basically correct and I believed, as did most of my colleagues, that the system was moving in the right direction.

It did not work out that way. The cost-cutters in our insurance companies were out to block all referrals to expensive specialists, often compelling the primary-care physicians to treat or manage things best left to specialists.

We will cover all these changes in subsequent chapters. Stay tuned.

Chapter 2: You Get What You Pay For

"the buck stops... where?"

Chapter summary: This chapter summarizes health care costs during the twentieth century, how they evolved, and the plusses and minuses of each step.

Until the 1950s, the patient was a customer in a pay-as-you-go system. Patients "bought" only a minimal amount of health care and checked the price of services very carefully. They changed doctors when the fees were too high, and hospitals were only a last resort. For the next 30 years or so, private and government health insurance programs developed, essentially reaching a point where they paid for all health care. Eventually patients began to demand more and more **("Spare no expense, doctor; I want the best")**. Doctors, facing an open cookie jar, offered more and more health care and kept patients in hospitals for longer and longer periods.

When the money ran out, managed care stepped in. At first, it put a great spin on what it was offering: quality assurance, a return to the primary-care doctor who knew his or her patients so well, and the elimination of useless and wasteful services. It was heaven on earth for insurance company number crunchers, who began using quality assurance as a pretext for rationing health care.

What we have today is "damaged" care or "mismanaged" care. For the system to improve, patients have to begin taking charge. They have to take the handcuffs off the doctors and stick them on the people who are rationing medical care.

Let's step back and take a bird's eye view of health care costs and how they have been covered in the United States during the 20th century. The issue is so complex that we could devote a whole book to it. I prefer to avoid all the nuances and to tell you how health care costs directly affect you as a patient.

Fee for Service: 1900-1950

The first half of the twentieth century relied essentially on the patient's wallet or pocketbook to pay for health care. A physician or a hospital offered a service, set a price, and then billed the patient. In some parts of the country a series of "gas" wars evolved, as doctors attempted to grab a larger and larger piece of the pie by lowering their prices. In other parts of the country price-fixing, now illegal, was set up by local medical societies. I recall such a fixed table of fees set by The Greater Lawrence Medical Society in Lawrence, Massachusetts, where my dad practiced medicine. Attached to his waiting room wall was a framed table of fees that enumerated the cost for a home visit, a telephone call, a series of routine operations, and on. In spite of the fixed fees, of course, doctors often negotiated their fees to capture more patients.

I like to call this "retail medicine" because it worked just like a retail store. You, the customer, enter a grocery store, for instance, and decide how many tomatoes, at what price, you need. You make all your choices based on price, your needs, and the quality of the goods. Your constraint is always the price tag, clearly listed on each product. Products may sell for roughly the same price in many stores or there may be real bargains here and there, provided you make the effort to look for them. Stores look for the cheapest source for their products and must always settle for only a reasonable profit. If they overcharge, the customer begins to walk away. Depending on demand and supply, stores come to understand the proper balance between profit and sales.

Free Service: 1950-1980

In the late '40s Blue Cross and Blue Shield came into existence and got involved with the doctors and hospitals in what was then called a cost-reimbursement arrangement. Putting aside all the little legalisms, it boiled down to the fact that the doctors and hospitals would set their rates and the insurance systems would pay them exactly what they asked. When Medicare and Medicaid began in 1965, the same cost reimbursement systems applied.

At first, neither the patients nor the doctors took unfair advantage of this neat arrangement. Patients went to doctors as they had over the years, and doctors prescribed services according to their set rituals. **In time both patient and doctor realized that cost reimbursement was a large cookie jar filled with wonderful cookies!** Patients began to demand more and more medical services for more and more problems. "Spare no expense, doctor, I want the best" echoed through the land. Doctors, in turn, began to deliver increasingly complex services, some demanded by the increasing and expensive technology, and some brought about simply because the insurance money was there for the asking. Hospitals were filled, expanded their services and offered all kinds of wonderful things to their happy in-patients.

The unintended consequence of cost-reimbursement or first-dollar insurance coverage was to inflate the demand for services by the patient and to inflate the meeting of that demand by the physician. It was said, often in jest but with some wisdom, that patients "purchased" health care up to the level of their insurance coverage and doctors delivered that care up to the level of the insurance coverage. At the same time, malpractice litigation increased by quantum leaps during the twenty-five years following the Second World War, and this led to extremely defensive, expensive medicine on the part of doctors. They ordered many tests, consulted with many specialists, and made greater and greater use of hospitalization—often to keep from being sued.

Flee From Service: 1980 to the present

By the early '80s the cookie jar began to empty. Employers resisted further increases in insurance costs to meet the increasing demands for services brought about by insurance coverage in the first place. Medicare was running out of funds, also due to overuse of services by patients, physicians, and hospitals. In addition, the public was becoming outraged with the proliferation of more and more expensive superspecialists in a system where the right hand did not know what the left hand was doing. Physicians did not communicate with each other very much, and the specialties led to a splintering of care.

It was time for some response. Federal legislation attempted to control the rising cost of care by requiring hospitals and labs to obtain federal permission before setting up competing treatment centers. In addition, they attempted to control the length of stay in hospitals by assigning physician bureaucrats to monitor the number of days in the hospital for each disease entity. These laws failed to contain rising costs.

Finally, some control of rising Medicare expenses came about when the government grouped all diseases into diagnosis related groups (DRGs) and paid fixed sums to hospitals for the management of these diseases. If the hospitals spent less than the allowed sum, they kept the difference. If they spent more, it showed up as hospital red ink. The government did the same with Medicare reimbursement of physicians, and the stage was set for the beginning of managed care, a private enterprise system brought about by health maintenance organizations and health insurance companies. Together they began to set fixed fees, lower the fees for services rendered and control when specialists could be called in by a primary care doctor.

It all sounded too good to be true. The clever spin-doctors from the government and the marketing experts from health maintenance organizations and health insurance companies heralded this new system as the end of duplicated services, the return of the primary-care physician to his or her rightful dominance of the health care system, and the end of confusion for the public. On and on went the spin.

What really was evolving was a system of rationing of health care by creating more and more roadblocks between the patient and his or her physicians. It became more and more difficult to communicate with them, more and more difficult to see a specialist, and hospital stays became dangerously shorter and shorter as HMOs, under the gun of insurance systems, forced patients out of the hospitals at times very prematurely in the judgment of many physicians, including me.

I choose to call this *flee from service.* Furthermore, the system of HMOs stood for *Heath Maintenance Organizations* but I prefer to call them ***Handcuffed Maintenance Organizations*** for that is what they have done to our physicians in an attempt to ration expensive health care. Throughout this book, I will show you how you can learn to manage this problem and help unfasten your doctors' handcuffs.

This "damaged" care or "mismanaged" care, as many have referred to it, exists up to the present time and, as I suggested in this chapter, patients must begin to take charge of things and handcuff the rationers of care.

Time Out!

Are there any solutions?

I am suggesting here that there are problems with each system: **fee, free, flee.**

Do I have a good answer to this dilemma? Should we totally reject our current managed care system? If so, do we return to fee-for-service or free service, and how do we solve the problems created by these two systems?

Is there a fourth option sitting out there in fantasyland, waiting to be discovered by someone brighter than I?

I do not have a clear answer. I ask you, the reader, to think about this issue as you peruse the chapters of this book. Just don't take any news media critic too seriously when he or she proposes a "simple solution" such as a national health care system. Each system has its strengths and its weaknesses, as I hope you will see as you give this more thought.

Chapter 3: What is a Primary or Personal Physician?

"the buck stops...here"

Chapter summary: The primary-care physician is like an orchestra conductor, whereas the specialist is like a member of the band, trained as a violinist or pianist or what have you. The primary physician is in charge of the whole health scene of his or her patient. This cannot be the responsibility of specialized physicians who know only one part of the human body and far less about the overall health of their patients.

Much of what the GP did was embodied, with some fanciful embellishments, in the Marcus Welby television series forty years ago. Welby, like the physician of old, cared for his patients in a very special way and offered them a sense of professional permanence, a continuity of care. He seemed comfortable treating the majority of human illnesses. When a specialist was needed, Dr. Welby considered himself responsible for seeking him out, while remaining the anchorman. There is security in knowing that your medical team has a captain or a manager, the job Dr. Welby did so well. He acted as a go-between, a sort of contact man between the patient and the specialist. He put in plain English what the specialist was saying, and reduced the whole complex arrangement to a workable, human, and intensely personal operation. In effect, Welby created a logical and rational system for his patients without depersonalizing medical care. **Welby was a primary-care physician.**

We have eliminated the primary-care physician, the general practitioner of old, and made no substitute. We have assumed, with disastrous effects, that all medicine needs is a series of high-powered specialists to cover each area of the human body, one piece at a time. As on a checkerboard, we have covered all the black spaces with our specialists but left just as many white spaces unprotected. The result is a hodgepodge of ever-multiplying and specialized physicians who, as a group, refuse to consider the whole patient their responsibility. Someone works on John Smith's middle ear and someone else checks his diabetes; someone worries about his marital troubles and someone else his gallbladder. But no one considers John Smith, who does not look upon his medical problems as limited to a painful gallbladder or an aching middle ear. Specialists might diagnose **disease** but it takes a committed primary care physician, interested in the patient and his entire family, to manage **dis-ease**.

A primary-care physician renders total patient care. That does not mean he does everything. It means simply that he is responsible for getting everything done. Specialists pass the patient, bucket-brigade fashion, from one to another, none feeling responsible for the whole patient.

Total patient care implies more. It suggests that the three phases of medical care—preventive, curative and rehabilitative—occupy the primary-care physician's time and effort. Specialists are just not capable of delivering such care. Preventive and rehabilitative medicine require a full knowledge of the personality of each patient, her living habits, her dietary and other indiscretions, and her family and social relationships. Here is where continuous care becomes so important. Of what real value is it to treat a patient for a moderately threatening acute illness, such as pneumonia, and pay no attention to the fact that he drinks and smokes too much, drives his car like a madman, overeats, and spends his work hours in a state of severe chronic tension? These factors must be considered by any physician who wants to prevent as well as treat disease. The technologically-oriented and overspecialized physician, caught up in his small area of expertise, tends to deride the value of preventive medicine, feeling it is something a counselor should be doing, not a physician.

Preventive medicine is the great challenge of the day. Technology has made the specialist's job quite easy by allowing us to turn over a greater and greater part of the diagnosis of disease to technicians. The big problem is prevention, for this requires that the physicians get their patients to comply with regimens that can bring a healthier life. It will require a primary-care physician working over the years to accomplish the job.

Rehabilitative medicine is also the province of the primary-care physician. It cannot be done adequately by the specialist. The cardiologist may be called in to advise and treat a patient with an acute heart attack. But rehabilitation is a lifelong proposition. It involves much more than a few pills and some heart exercise. It requires a lifetime program of re-education for the coronary-prone patient. He must adopt a new life-style if he is to avoid another catastrophic and possibly fatal heart attack. The entire living pattern of this patient must be radically and permanently altered for success in this phase of medicine. After the cardiologist does his or her thing in management of the acute phase of the heart attack, the primary-care physician takes over the rehabilitative phase of the patient's life.

The transient relationship between a patient and a specialist makes this task impossible. But a primary-care or personal physician sees his patients regularly. He can remind them that a change in diet is necessary, that nicotine is a cardiac killer, that reasonable exercise is salutary, that work tensions must be avoided, and so on.

A primary-care physician is in a position to develop a personal, intimate relationship with his patients. One way to do this is the home visit. I would like to see home visits evolve as part of the normal pattern for a primary physician. Like my dad, I hasten to distinguish the home visit from a house call. There is rarely anything to be gained by returning to the grossly inefficient house call. The physician cannot render valid medical service for an acute illness with the few gadgets and pills there is room for in his black bag. Modern Medicine requires that the ailing patient come to the hospital, clinic or doctor's office where special equipment is available.

But a home visit is something else again. I am thinking here of an annual social visit that a physician would make to each of his families. It would permit the physician to see his patients in the context of their family situation. While it may not uncover some of the subtle psychological forces at work, the whole milieu of the family situation will present itself. The nutritional state of the children, basic hygiene habits and health hazards may be discovered by the physician. These may help him understand episodic illnesses occurring in the family.

The home visit would also reduce the professional barriers that separate a doctor from her patients. I think the physician should become a friend of each of her patients and not keep herself separate from them by the pomp and circumstance of her profession and the artificial barriers induced by the sterile atmosphere of her office. There is no doubt in my mind that the house call served this purpose quite well.

The great suburban sprawl has made the home visit a very difficult concept. To ask physicians to find their way into each patient's home for the annual home visit may be impossible. Suffice to say, much has been lost and perhaps can never be regained again. It is, however, worth the try!

A primary-care physician, then, is one who practices continuous, total patient care, preventive, curative, and rehabilitative in a very personal, intimate way. This is the type of physician I recommend to you. If your present physician falls short of this, you should re-evaluate your choices.

Time Out!

Home visit? Primary care? Spending time with patients? Knowing the entire medical history of a patient?

Time out indeed! So long as third parties control the dispensation of monies to pay for health care, the physicians will be handcuffed and a true relationship between a primary-care physician and his or her patient cannot exist. **The kind of relationship I am describing in this book becomes pure fantasy**.

Is there any hope? Indeed there is. Slowly but surely the public is beginning to cast off HMO medicine and managed care. The whole point of this book is to make you aware of the damaging effects of managed care and insurance-controlled medicine so that you can state your case strongly and boldly whenever you visit a physician handcuffed by number crunchers and rationing agents of insurance companies or government health bureaucracies.

You will be amazed if not shocked with how quickly these systems react and cave in once you become knowledgeable about the rationing game they are playing and you demand more personal care.

Chapter 4: How Not to Choose a Doctor

"pay no attention to the man behind the screen"

Chapter Summary: This chapter examines methods that people use to choose a doctor, including the prestige of his or her medical school, the board certification plaque in the waiting room, or what a hospital administrator has to say about the doctor. These methods are either totally impractical or simply factitious.

Quality is a very difficult thing to measure. The vast majority of American medical school graduates are qualified and intelligent, but these characteristics do not guarantee good medical care. There's far more to it than that.

The issue is whether the doctor has heart.

The idea of writing this book came to me over the years as I listened, amused and amazed, to people discuss how they choose their doctors. I must credit government, consumer-advocacy groups and the news media for making some people conscious of the need to make a choice. This is more than I can say for Organized Medicine which has remained completely silent over the years.

The problem with government and various consumer-advocacy groups is that they are hung up on the phrase **"quality of medical care."** You hear and read it all over the place. It sounds great. Who can possibly be against such a noble idea and such a laudable enterprise: "Improve the quality of medical care."

Unfortunately, quality is an extremely difficult concept to define, measure or recognize. It means many different things to different people. It implies that we've all agreed on the goals or purposes of medical care and only have to see how our present system measures up to those goals.

But have we really settled on anything? What is the goal, for example, of cancer therapy? Is it to prolong the life of an individual as long as possible? If so, those treatments that yield the highest longevity statistics would be defined as high quality. Or perhaps the goal is to prolong useful, comfortable life? Then quality is measured in far different ways. Is the goal of a good cardiologist limited to lowering the mortality of the coronary victim, or is it to rehabilitate him or to prevent him from having the coronary in the first place? Perhaps the goal includes all three or some other objective not yet recognized.

Cadillac or Corvette?

I do not believe the concept "quality of medical care" is ever going to be concrete enough to yield a meaningful measure by which you can choose a good doctor. It's like asking, "which is the higher-quality car, a Cadillac or Corvette?" It all depends on what you want to get out of a car in the first place.

"Quality of care" may have value to the academicians but I am interested in setting down practical, concrete criteria that you can use in choosing a good physician. Some will say this can't be done because the public is not scientifically trained and is therefore incapable of deciding what is good medicine or who is a good doctor. That is an elitist view—one that I totally reject. Given the proper orientation, you are capable of deciding whether or not your doctor is a good one. Furthermore, you and only you can make this judgment. In the final analysis you must be satisfied about your relationship with your doctor, and no one else can tell you how to measure that value. That is why free choice is so important and must be maintained. Any system that compels you to accept Dr. X. rather than Dr. Y simply to make the system work is deceptive, precisely because personal satisfaction is such an individual thing and an essential part of the healing process. **Beware the mismanaged care of HMOs and insurance companies who try to limit your choice.**

Ways To Choose a Doctor

Where do we begin? Let's start by considering several ways of choosing a doctor that don't work. A frequent suggestion—I'm sure you've read it in popular magazines—is to check the medical school your physician attended. The theory is simple but useless: if he went to a good school, he must be good; if to a bad school he must be bad. This myth had some validity seventy-five years ago when dozens of half-baked medical schools flourished in the United States. Fortunately these schools have been eliminated. All medical schools in this country are fully accredited and offer students a high-quality education.

What about the distinction between Ivy League schools and all the rest? **An Ivy League education is no guarantee that its graduates are any better than graduates of less prestigious, but fully accredited, medical schools.**

What about checking the physician's board certification? The specialty boards were created to certify that their members have completed an approved residency and are qualified to practice that specialty. Board certification is a minimum standard of excellence. If your specialist does not have his boards, be very cautious in dealing with him. But if he does, you still have no guarantee that he's a good doctor. Since the majority of physicians have their boards, you're back with the same dilemma. Everybody seems well qualified on paper but incompetency still flourishes. You must constantly keep in mind this principle: **Paper certification does not produce professional excellence.** No matter how many degrees a doctor has, how many pieces of paper claiming expertise in this or that branch of medicine, his performance is what counts and that is not measured by report cards.

Then there are those who will advise you to contact your local medical society when choosing a doctor. This is an absurd suggestion and a complete waste of your time. Local medical societies are not set up to be referral agencies and, at best, will give you a list of all physicians in your area with no comment about which are good, which bad.

How about calling your local hospital? That's been suggested and I mention it only to denounce it. They'll simply tell you the names of physicians who have staff privileges—about the same list as in the yellow pages. A hospital staff is not a judge of the individual physician. Staff privileges are granted to all physicians who apply, providing they fulfill a minimum number of qualifications, such as a state licensure and board certification. Once on a staff, physicians must be treated equally by the hospital and any effort to steer patients to this or that physician is considered quite inappropriate. Besides, what about the competency of those doing the steering?

Some consumer groups publish guidebooks which list local physicians plus a profile of their working arrangements, their fees, the number of hours they spent in postgraduate education, whether they are board certified, and so on. These are useless as guides to quality care or professional excellence. To the extent that they tell you what hours a doctor sees patients and something about his fees they may be useful. But they are totally deceiving when they claim to measure excellence.

Believe me, they do no such thing. They are based on surveys made by calling doctors and asking them to list their credentials, what courses they have taken, which journals they read, and what meetings they attend. Assuming that each physician answers the questionnaire with absolute honesty, what in the world does the information prove? So Dr. A attends fourteen post-graduate and Dr. B only eight. Dr. A, as it turns out, also reads eight medical journals a month, while Dr. B reads only four. But that does not mean Dr. A is a better physician than Dr. B.

Certificates do not Equal Excellence

The basic principle is simple: No amount of documentation with medical credentials says a thing about professional excellence. You just cannot measure the QUALITY of human service by QUANTITATIVE means.

All these suggestions for choosing a good doctor are based on the tenuous premise that a piece of paper, such as a diploma or board certificate, a survey of courses taken, or a document stating a doctor serves on a hospital medical staff, guarantees that he or she is a good doctor. Unfortunately, all modern doctors look good on paper. They all have licenses, all have some certifying statement, all belong to one or more medical societies, almost all have hospital privileges, and all respond to consumer surveys in a way best calculated to show their good side. All these methods for choosing a doctor are based on a false premise: namely, that an informed doctor is a good doctor. The best you can say about a well-informed doctor is that, given a multiple-choice test about medical science, he tends to get a gold star. The problem is that medical science must be applied to the ailing human and that takes more than a well-informed medical scientist.

Nor do any of these methods screen out the lemons in the medical profession. They are usually quite adept at looking good on paper. They have good survival qualities! Lacking competency, they develop a variety of "look-good" mechanisms, not the least of which is to join half a dozen medical organizations that make no demands on competency but issue nicely framed and fancy-sounding certificates for $100 a year. They may look good but hardly satisfy your need and quest for excellence. Lists of "good" and "bad" doctors found on the web, lists you are often required to pay for, talk only about outright failures, characteristics that usually show up in malpractice courts and are only a negative mark, saying nothing about who are the good doctors.

Is this an excessively cynical view? I do not think so. Bear in mind that there is a tremendous selection process in the pursuit of a medical career. It is a long and arduous course of study and only top-notch students with great staying power get through the system. Those who make it, for whatever reason, are well qualified on paper and have an excellent education. But that doesn't make them excellent physicians and that is the rub. Whatever it takes to turn a well-informed medical scientist into a humane, considerate and responsible physician with a balanced judgment and a correct set of priorities cannot be measured by objective standards. **The heart of the matter is heart—that is what separates the excellent physician from the mediocre.**

Time Out!

"Pay No Attention to the Man Behind the Screen." These critical words, defining the moment of truth for the Wizard of Oz, are more real than Dorothy's fantasy could ever imagine.

I feel like a prophet when I re-read this chapter written twenty years ago about how quality is so difficult to measure. National quality assurance committees (QA) of the JOINT COMMISSION FOR THE ACCREDITATION OF HOSPITALS have changed their name to the enfeebled concept *quality improvement* or QI. They have dropped the term ***quality assurance*** (QA) because they know darn well they cannot assure quality.

Distortions of Mass Marketing

If diplomas and other paper certifications were not good ways to judge quality in 1980, where do things stand today? Like the man behind the screen, the Wizard's reputation proved nothing then and is far more tenuous today. In this era of Health Maintenance Organizations (HMOs), mass marketing has distorted the situation beyond any certifying agency's ability to find and measure and guarantee quality. **HMO administrations and health insurance companies are very adept at clever, self-serving and often distorted advertising**. When it was only the doctor and his yellow pages, it might be easy to flesh out the phony ads; not so with clever modern marketing which uses real professionals and a great deal of cash to promote so-called high quality doctors and health institutions. The yellow pages have multi-colored ads, billboards sing the praises of this or that specialty group, television space is increasingly devoted to showing you good service and high quality professionalism. There are web sites that sing the praises of this or that group of docs.

As physicians become more specialized and more and more associated with large groups, the idea that a diploma hanging on a doctor's office wall can help you pick quality is a sham. Some diplomas represent significant accomplishments. More often than not, however, he or she has strung a host of diplomas and certificates from this or that medical organization all over the office wall. It becomes almost impossible to see the wallpaper after a while. These certificates often represent rather hollow medical societies that, in effect, sell these diplomas for hanging on a doctor's wall. In other instances the medical organization in question is legitimate but requires no credentials other than a valid medical license to be a member. These societies do not in any way represent quality symbols for doctors.

If the Wizard of Oz was exposed as a little less that magical by the facts of the case, recall also that the diploma hung around the tin man's chest, giving him a college diploma and making him smart, was just that, a product of fantasy gone awry. The movie glamorized the tin man. It made us all feel good. We must not settle for such fiction when it comes to our physicians. I pray and believe physicians are more important to you than Dorothy's tin man.

All the great and expensive marketing in the world created by HMOs and health insurance companies do not change this fact, learned a long time ago: **Diplomas and other paper certificates of excellence make great wallpaper, nothing more, often something less.**

Chapter 5: How to Begin Your Search

"can you hear the smile in her voice?"

Chapter summary: This chapter introduces you to the idea that you must make a real choice over physicians. People shop around before buying a car. When it comes to who will take care of them in health and disease, some seem to think it all works automatically. Others develop very convoluted means for choosing a doctor. A patient who lives in a small suburb many miles from a major city somehow desires to have a "prestigious" doctor at a "prestigious" medical center. He makes that arrangement, sees the top-notch, a-number-1 rated doctor three times while he is well and then, late at night a critical emergency hits him and he is forced to seek attention at his local hospital by a physician who does not know him at all.

Here I put a practical focus on beginning your search. It is only a beginning and much has to be done after the initial and tentative choice is made.

If you are the type who buys a car at first glance or an expensive camera on casual recommendation of one friend, skip this chapter as it will turn you off. **But if choice is vital, as it should be when picking a physician, then please pay careful attention to what I am saying here.** Take notes; even better, underline the ideas and talk them over with your spouse, friends or relatives.

Here are the four major factors you must consider when choosing a physician:

1. **Define your bias: Some people are happy when they have chosen a physician close to home. Others are never secure unless their physicians are attached to major teaching institutions in our big cities. Don't fight this bias; it will always haunt you, especially if you choose a doctor counter to the bias and something (not necessarily his or her fault) goes wrong.**
2. **Know your physical limitations: Age is an important one, as are any known physical or psychological illnesses from which you suffer. These often demand that your doctors be located very close to your residence. Be realistic about these limitations.**
3. **Be conscious of your travel accommodations: Do you drive a car? Must others take you to your doctor? If so, what are their calendar limitations?**
4. **What are your geographical limitations? How far are you willing to travel for routine and emergency medical care? How long will it take you to get to your doctor or your hospital? What is the traffic flow from your home to his or her office or the hospital?**

Let's explore all this in greater detail. Take what I am saying seriously but not religiously. If you have better ideas or if some of this does not appeal, that is fine. Give some thought to what I am saying, as it is based on three decades of studying this problem of choice. Modify it according to your best judgment but do so with some reservation.

What type of doctor should you look for? I strongly recommend that you limit your search to primary-care physicians, avoiding specialists. Look for an internist or a family physician.

Your search should have certain geographic limitations, usually determined by where you live, what highways are accessible, where the hospitals are located, and so on. Don't become an itinerant patient, seeking your primary medical care in far off places simply because the "big city offers so much more." It just isn't so. Most physicians feel perfectly secure being treated by colleagues in their own communities. The lure of big city specialists (unless, of course, you live in a big city) is often impractical and sometimes dangerous. If a real crisis arises you'll need to find the nearest emergency room. How much better for you if you are able to call upon a physician who knows you well. The "big city" may be too far away when emergencies arise. If there are physicians in your community who are accepting patients, try one of them, reserving big city physicians for those few occasions when your local doctor recommends them. **But always remain true to your bias. Don't swallow my bias, hook, line and sinker. If "prestigious" conjures up magical powers for you, then go for the "prestigious."**

If you drive, your perimeters will be wider, but the closer to home the physician's office the better. Ideally your social life will mix with that of your doctor. A generation ago the family doctor was a member of a nearby church, joined various social clubs and, along with his patients, took part in town and civic activities. Such communal living fostered greater mutual loyalty and lifelong bonds and trust that are almost impossible today. Sprawling suburban communities, frequent job relocations and a far more rapid pace of living have destroyed these bonds. Choosing a doctor in your community may help to re-create some of this mutual respect.

Take what I am saying seriously but not religiously.

Beginning your search:

One way to begin your search, and it is only a preliminary step, is to use the yellow pages. Turn to them for a list of primary-care physicians available in your community. Copy their names in a notebook. Let us assume your community has eight internists and four family doctors. Place their names along with their addresses and telephone numbers in your notebook.

Go to your local library and ask for the AMA Physician's Directory. It will give you important information about these twelve doctors and help you in your choice.

Age: A physician's age can be an important factor in your choice. Cultural and communication differences do exist and can be age-related even though this may sound politically incorrect. Check your list and eliminate physicians on the retirement side of things.

Board Certification: This is a minimum standard for choosing a good doctor. There are exceptions, but to be on the right side of the law of averages you should choose a board-certified internist or family practitioner. Checking your list again, eliminate those who do not have their boards.

Your list gets shorter and shorter as you consider age, certification and location. This is only a start; you have a long, long way to go.

There is nothing further to be gained from the Physician's Directory. It will tell you each doctor's premedical and medical school education, as well as various specialty societies he belongs to. This information will not help you make your choice.

This exercise assumes a small community with only a few potential physicians to choose from. The list could get unwieldy if it got much beyond forty or fifty doctors but that should immediately suggest that you have not defined your perimeters carefully and are wandering all over the map. So if your list is long, take a closer look at where their offices are, how accessible they are, what traffic is like during the busy shopping hours, what kind of parking facilities there are, and so on. Such considerations may seem trivial, but if you can find a good doctor conveniently located why not do so?

Next, ask friends about the doctors on your list. (I'm going to talk about reputation in the next chapter.) Be sure you ask a good number of people, but don't draw conclusions too quickly from what they tell you. In the final analysis, only you will be able to judge which of these physicians best suits your needs and which are really good doctors. But a few preliminary inquiries will do no harm.

Some of the things you might want to ask are as follows:

- Is the physician easy to talk to? Does he use "big words" to gratify his ego?
- How accessible is he? What is his coverage system? What docs work with him?
- How expensive?
- How reliable does she seem?
- Is her office easy to reach?
- What about parking?
- How long do you wait in her waiting room? Does she keep most appointments?

- Does he have evening office hours?
- Does he have hospital privileges? Where are these hospitals located?
- Does he refer often to other specialists or does he frown on second opinions?

The next step: call each of these doctors. Chances are you'll speak with the receptionist. Introduce yourself; tell him or her that you're looking for a new physician. Don't be discouraged if you're told the doctor is not taking new patients. Often this means for the time being. Tell the receptionist that you're in no rush (you've planned ahead), that you're not ill at present, and that you would like to make an appointment for whenever the doctor has time.

Ask about his or her appointment schedule and fees for services. Don't be shy about talking money. This usually means to the secretary that you're conscientious about paying doctors' bills and simply wish to find out if the fees are within the limitations of your pocketbook.

Try to pick up the tone of the receptionist's voice. Her method of dealing with patients quite often reflects her boss's attitude. If she's friendly, warm, and takes time with you, her boss will probably be the same. If she's brusque, cold, and shuts you off abruptly, beware.

Combining your discussion with friends and your telephone interviews, you can narrow the choice further. One or more of the doctors may not be seeing new patients under any condition. One may not enjoy a very good reputation among several of your friends. That leaves a few from whom to make your preliminary choice. If your final list is longer, ten to twenty physicians, for example, start with those that seem most accessible.

Time Out!

Two decades of suburban sprawl, transient living as we change jobs a dozen times in a lifetime, the convenience of cellular phones, and the grouping of doctors in larger and larger building complexes have made many a dent in the yellow page ritual which I described above. In short, we no longer live in quaint, "good morning, how are you Bill" neighborhoods where we knew everyone and they knew us. It might have been a simpler world, but modernism has also brought with it a greater power to cure in the hands of our physicians.

The yellow pages have not become outmoded, provided you use them **only as a very first step**. They can give you a few facts about the doctors' locations in your area and nothing more.

The phone call inquiring about the doctor will tell you much more than his or her schedule. When you make those inquiring calls, pay particular attention to the following parameters. These were not important issues when I first wrote the book as most offices had one telephone receptionist and it was a rather easy way of getting through. With the dawn of large group practices and HMOs, getting through to the office is a headache in itself.

So here are things to look for:

1. Does the receptionist answer the phone for one or more doctors? "Hello, Dr. Wallace's office; thank you for calling; how may I help you?" Or, "Good afternoon, Drs. Jones, Smith, Holiday and Laxity's office: how may we help you?"
2. Does the receptionist answer the phone or does an answering service intervene? If it is an answering service, call at different times to see if there is ever a receptionist answering the phone.
3. If you reach a receptionist, what is her or his level of politeness and desire to accommodate you? This is a key feature and is not likely to change as time goes on. The person answering the phone may be the most critical person in your relationship with the physician. Never underestimate the importance of a good, open, helpful receptionist. Further, it is a real safe bet that she reflects her boss's attitudes. **Listen carefully: what you want to "hear" is a smile in her voice.**
4. Let me give an example of this from my own practice: I happened to overhear a phone discussion between a patient calling in and a receptionist whom I had just hired. Let us call the receptionist Mary. I only heard her side of the conversation but I could easily surmise what had transpired.
   The call came in after a rather busy day, at about 5 p.m.

"Hello," Mary said, "can I help you?"

After a pause, during which time the patient had apparently explained the reason for her call, she being a new patient calling for the first time, I heard Mary say:

"Gee no; I am sorry Ma'am. Dr. LeMaitre is a surgeon and does not take care of chest pain."

There was some further remark or two, unimportant for this illustration, and then Mary hung up.

"What was that all about, Mary," I inquired.

"Oh just some old lady with chest pain."

"Where was she from?"

"I didn't ask, Dr. LeMaitre, why?"

I asked Mary to call back. The patient lived five minutes from our office. The chest pain was mild. I instructed my secretary to inform the patient that I was a surgeon, that I would check her briefly and refer her to a primary-care doctor **and there would be no charge**.

I examined her. I called a primary-care doctor and referred the lady for an examination. She was grateful for that service. I also knew the primary-care doctor would be grateful for receiving a new patient and he would surely pay me back someday with a surgical referral.

"You see, Mary" I explained, "everyone gains in this way: the patient does not feel rejected, the primary-care doctor receives a new patient and, for sure, I will be rewarded both with a sense of service and perhaps a patient at a later date."

I was not comfortable that Mary really understood. She seemed resentful. I listened carefully over the next few weeks. Things did not improve. She had an instinct for getting to "no" with patients. I insist that my people always get to "yes." I had to let her go.

And you must pay careful heed to the receptionist and be sure she gets to "yes" whenever you chat with her.

Let me make this very concrete. You are calling for the first time. It is not an emergency; you simply wish to see if the doctor is taking new patients, something about his charges, what insurance he takes and when you might see him or her.

I am going to give you extreme cases; often the real world is not so definite, but I wish you to get a clear message about the difference and how some receptionists always manage to get to "no" and others always find a way to get to "yes." In this illustration the doctor is unable to see you for about twelve weeks. Your name is Mary Smith.

1. The receptionist getting to "no":

"Hello, my name is Mary Smith. I am calling to find out if Dr. Jones is taking new patients. This is not an emergency but I want to set up an appointment for a full examination."

"Well I am not at my work station so I don't have doctor's appointment book with me. He's pretty busy for the next several months. Why don't you try again at the end of the summer? Doctor is taking no new cases until then."

You can plug in any number of such negative responses from secretaries **who sound like they have a toothache when you first call them**.

Keep in mind that the receptionist is the first keeper at the gate whenever you have a medical problem and she is not likely to get any better as time goes on.

2. The receptionist getting to "yes":

"Hello my name is Mary Smith. I am new in town and looking for a primary-care physician. Is Dr. Jones taking new patients"?

"Hello Mary, my named is Karen Albright. I am Dr. Jones' receptionist. Thank you for calling. Hold on a moment Mary, I'll get our appointment book and see what we can do. (pause) Here we are; sorry to keep you waiting. Gosh the very next routine appointment I have here is twelve weeks from Tuesday. Mary, do you feel this can wait or is there some emergency? If so we can fit you in for a quick visit to check that out and then bring you back later for a full exam? (pause) Okay I am glad things aren't urgent so we will see you on Tuesday, August 14 at 11 a.m. We'll send you a note confirming the appointment. If anything more urgent occurs, Mary, please give us a call. Just ask to speak to me, Karen. (pause) Thank you so much for calling. Bye now."

Don't be in a rush to accept an appointment with the first doctor who is able to give you one. Write down the date but make a couple of phone calls each day. You can always cancel them all before the dates are reached. Keep a close ear to the offices with receptionists who get to "no" and mark these down as strong negatives as you add up the pros and cons of this early search for the right doctor.

I can tell you after thirty years of dealing with doctors and their receptionists that in the long run you will be a very wise patient if you steadfastly avoid the doctor whose receptionist gets to "no" when you talk with her. Observe this rule. **Those secretaries getting to "no" and those getting to "yes" are remarkably consistent. They don't change from time to time and you cannot really ever correct the bad ones**. They are not malicious; they hardly know what good customer service means. They just don't get it and should be avoided at all costs.

I was unable to change the negative attitude of my new secretary. Bear in mind I was her boss, the guy who paid her salary, and I could not make her answer the phone with a smile in her voice and a "yes" in her responses. It is unlikely that you will do any better with that secretary who could not find her appointment book for you. My advice: stay clear of her and her physician boss. It will only make you sicker to deal with her.

Chapter 6: Can You Rely on a Doctor's Reputation?

"round up the usual suspects"

Chapter summary: This chapter begins the slow, steady process by which you begin to choose the good doctor. Just as you choose a new car by looking at the standard makes and avoiding the Mongrel Car Company, you must begin your search for a good doctor by checking out the reputation of doctors in your hometown. It's only a start and there will be many, many more steps to take but **begin with reputation**. The restaurant with the filled parking lot is likely to be a good restaurant.

I submit that one of the best places to begin in choosing a doctor is with his reputation. Doctors who enjoy good reputations are very likely to be good doctors.

It is so important for you to understand what a good reputation is that I must digress for a moment and take you back seventy years or so when reputation had no validity whatsoever. People were easily taken in by quacks. The quack was a smooth-sounding, affable, "solid citizen" who made an art out of reputation-building but had little professional competency. Some people are still charmed by the smart sounding doctor, which is why **you cannot choose your doctor on the strength of a neighbor's suggestion alone.**

People are more sophisticated now. The mystique of medicine is rapidly disappearing and the public is far less apt to be fooled by the charlatan. Thus, a good reputation, based on widespread acceptance, is a valid criterion of a good doctor.

As you ask around about doctors—at work, at church, at cocktail parties—the same names will come up again and again. Look for consensus. If you keep your eyes and ears open, you will soon know which doctors enjoy good reputations. It may take several weeks, but it's worth the time and effort.

Have you noticed how often busy restaurants turn out to be the good ones? People seek excellence. The same is true with doctors. Reputations are built on excellence and people have an uncanny way of recognizing it. You will rarely go wrong by sticking to the principle that **reputation follows excellence**.

Let me illustrate. Several years ago, while vacationing in a small town miles from home, one of my children became ill. I did not wish to treat a member of my family. Realizing the importance of choosing the best doctor I could under these unusual circumstances, I stepped into a local bank and asked to speak with the President. My guess was that he would be reasonably astute and not likely to be fooled by charlatans. I was using the principle of reputation. Lacking time, I was unable to get a variety of opinions. I asked what pediatrician he would recommend. He was amused that I was asking him. I'm sure he's still wondering about it and entertaining his friends with the tale.

Well, why not? It's as good a place to start and, in a pinch, it beats meaningless lists of names from a hospital administrator who is ethically forbidden to steer patients to the good doctors.

When I took my daughter to the pediatrician, I pointed out that he had been highly recommended by the local banker and that, being somewhat anxious about a strange doctor, I was relieved to get such a highly respected doctor to see my child. I avoided telling him that I was a physician. A good doctor not only earns his reputation but is ennobled by it. Defending it makes him go the extra mile, even with a stranger. I was not only impressed with his performance but got my money's worth in the bargain.

Over the years, I have worked with some 1,000 doctors, 200 of whom have been flat tires, duds, or whatever you wish to label them, just bad doctors. **With strikingly few exceptions, most of this 20 percent did not enjoy good reputations**. Conversely, the top-notch physicians I worked with had excellent reputations.

Whether you are the police sergeant in the classic film Casablanca ("rounding up the usual suspects") or a patient looking for a good doctor, reputation is what it is all about.

Reputation is only a start; you have a long, long way to go before placing your life or the life of your loved ones in the hands of a particular physician. Still, a good reputation is a good start provided you take your time in evaluating the judgment of others who are recommending a particular physician.

Once you have completed the basic steps in these first few chapters, you are ready to enter a doctor's office and begin the really substantial evidence gathering in your ongoing search for a good doctor.

Time Out!

It is true that people are more sophisticated about medical science today than 70 years ago when charlatans and scam artists roamed the medical world and took advantage of an uneducated, often illiterate public.

Still, charlatans today use very sophisticated methods. Often these are well-trained physicians that simply want to take advantage of the health insurance system by ordering unnecessary tests and doing unnecessary procedures on an unwary public. Given the fear that many diseases can raise, it is no wonder that patients are willing to undergo overblown exams at the mere suggestion that these tests might detect or prevent disease.

Good reputation alone cannot guarantee that your doctor does not order unnecessary tests. Indeed, he might gain support for these tests by a public that feels he is very thorough and conscientious.

There is another subtle scheme that some doctors use to encourage the belief that they enjoy an excellent reputation. Busy doctors, like busy restaurants, often imply high-quality care. Imagine getting an appointment to see Dr.X at 3 pm next Monday. You arrive and find a filled office, standing room only! "Goodness", you say to yourself, "this doctor must be excellent. He surely enjoys a good reputation. His office is jammed with patients."

Wait! Ask around; you may find that everyone there got a 3 p.m.appointment. This is called **appointment jamming**, a not-so-subtle but effective way to “prove” how busy and therefore excellent the doctor really is.

Appointment jamming is not a common practice but you must be aware of this possibility when you are out to judge a doctor’s reputation. That just goes to show you that **reputation alone does not a good doctor make**. There is much more that you have to discover before making that judgment.

One more caveat. Although, as I said, people are more sophisticated and less apt to be fooled by the charlatan than years ago, the newest entry into the “make doc look good” field is the commercialism surrounding many group practices and HMOs. They place a great deal of money and time and energy in the box marked “show how good our docs are” and you must be very careful about newspaper and tv and web site ads which tell you so many good things about their doctors. Just read on in this book and take plenty of notes.

Chapter 7: The Most Important Sign of a Good Doctor

"look before you keep"

Chapter summary: Curing begins and ends with caring; the two are inseparable. A good doctor first and foremost cares about his or her patients, and you can begin the process of figuring out if your new doctor cares about you by consciously running through a list that this chapter presents to you: how long you wait in the doctor's waiting room; how long is your visit; how carefully does he listen to your symptoms; how often does she interrupt your talk to speed you along, so-called "pacing the patient"; does he resist sending you for second opinions or referring you to another type of specialist? These and a hundred similar questions, gestures which you will learn to observe carefully, will tell you far more than certificates on his wall how good he is by how much he cares for you as a human being. Some doctors wear long, white coats and some just roll up their sleeves. Neither tells you what's inside or what's down deep in your new doctor. **Look for signs that he or she cares and you're on your way to a good choice**.

There you are in a new doctor's office. You've made your preliminary choice. Now, you're waiting to meet him. What's the most important sign of a good doctor—something that will tip you off that you've placed your life in competent hands?

Don't bother looking at those diplomas and certificates on the wall unless you're bored. They all say he's a grade A doctor.

They wouldn't be hanging there otherwise. They make good wallpaper (sometimes) but nothing else.

And don't be overly impressed if his nurse or medical secretary looks "professional." While important, it has little to do with the doctor's competency.

The most important sign of a good doctor is that he cares about you as a person. Your first visit should help you to sense this important sign, provided you keep it in mind and concentrate on his words and reactions. Begin by asking yourself how long he made you sit in his waiting room. There may be extenuating circumstances, such as an emergency. But did his receptionist apologize and explain the cause of the delay? Generally, he should work out his appointment schedule with your convenience in mind. If you've waited more than twenty minutes, you are justified in wondering whether he has any respect for your schedule. People who keep me waiting unduly, with no respect for my busy schedule, don't really care about me. They'll never go the extra mile to serve me, which makes me very nervous about any long-term relationship.

Whereas a busy physician is usually a good one, an over-scheduled physician can't help cutting corners. A physician who cares about his patients does not permit himself to be overextended just for the added economic gain. A good physician is extremely thorough and leaves no stone unturned. **Diagnosis and treatment are not magic tricks. They require time and hard work.** The over-busy doctor has compromised these requirements to make more money. He does not care enough about you to limit his practice to manageable numbers.

So what is his waiting room scene like? Is it a traffic jam, with people coming and going in large numbers? Watch the next few patients who go into his consulting or examining rooms. How long do they stay? If it's in and out, you should be alert for an assembly-line operation. It may seem efficient but that's not what good medicine is all about. A good physician deals with people who have problems, not just the problems themselves. Their illnesses are often quite obvious and not time-consuming for the doctor. Often it is the patient's lifestyle that is the key to his or her disease, and this takes time to figure out. A doctor who solves a patient's problems in a hurry, charges for them, and goes on to the next one, might be an efficient technician, but he doesn't really care about his patients. **Good medicine takes time.**

It's not easy to define "care" but good care is very easy to recognize. It's something you can sense and it is measured in little ways. Let's start negatively and examine the doctor who does not care about you. How can you recognize him?

Concentrate on his eye contact and his responses to your anecdotes about your health. You will soon be aware that he is putting on an act, letting you go through your little story of woe, hardly listening to you. He is tuned off, concentrating on moving you through quickly so he can get to his next patient.

I once saw a delightful cartoon about this kind of doctor. It depicted a psychiatrist, seated at his desk, seemingly concentrating on everything his patient was saying. His eyes, however, were aimed at a hidden television under his desk displaying a baseball game. He was able to stay in contact with his patient's monologue enough to offer an occasional, "Yes, of course. Go on," and still follow the course of the ball game. **Just a cartoon? I'm afraid not.**

Some doctors are very adept at keeping two such streams of consciousness running. They fool their patients only because no one has ever alerted the patients to look for the vacant stare, the lost thread of the conversation, the slightly irrelevant response to the question, and all the other telltale signs of a physician who really doesn't give a damn about the patient or his problems.

A doctor who does not care about you has a restless urge to interrupt your conversation, to cut you short and aim you in some other direction. He is pacing you, forcing you into his time frame. You can sense that he has a mental eye on the time clock, allotting you five or ten minutes.

A doctor who does not care will not permit irrelevancies in your conversation. If you happen to mention your work, one of your hobbies or interests, he will not pursue this with a follow-up question but will quickly return you to the medical conversation from which you momentarily departed.

There is, of course, another side to this story. Some patients are thoughtless windbags who wander from one subject to the other, seemingly unconscious that there are other patients waiting to be seen. This is a judgment that you will have to make about yourself. The fault may not be altogether the doctor's.

The doctor who cares exudes it from the moment you meet her. You can tell by the way she greets you, listens to what you have to say, and pursues your interests without pacing you. (This can be just an act, of course, but artificiality wears thin after a while. It may take one or two visits to see through the smile, but with attention you can sift out the phony.)

The doctor who cares is thorough, conscientious, quick to admit her own shortcomings, and honest enough to seek the help of specialists if she feels they can contribute to your well-being. She is loyal to her patients, following through on the minute details of good patient care, and is always available when you need her most.

Not long ago I bumped into a former patient at a social event. I had referred her and her husband to an internist for primary care. She praised me to the high heavens for introducing her to Dr. X, "the best damned doctor in town." Once I settled her down, I told her I was gratified that the referral had turned out so well and asked her why such admiration for Dr. X. She told me that her husband had been hospitalized and placed in the coronary care unit as a precautionary measure. Dr. X was on vacation and his partner took over management of the case. On his third day in the hospital, she recounted, Dr. X telephoned her husband in the coronary care unit. He said he was still on vacation, had heard from his partner that his patient had been admitted to the hospital, and just wanted to reassure him that everything was going fine. Apparently the partner, Dr. Y, had sensed that the wife felt a little anxious that Dr. X was not present for this first major illness. Therefore he called Dr. X and suggested that he call the patient and his wife just to reassure them.

Playing the devil's advocate, I attempted to deflate her enthusiasm for Dr. X (whom I most respect) by pointing out that she was praising him and he wasn't even around to take care of her husband. "**That's not the point, Doctor," she fired back. "If he cared enough to make that phone call, we're in good hands."**

There's more wisdom in those words than a skeptic's analysis might suggest. Caring for patients is not something one can turn on just to suit the customer. It cannot be programmed into a doctor by any form of education, certification, or licensing. It's an instinct that some doctors have and some haven't. It acts as a well-spring for the intellectual energies needed to practice good medicine.

I have never met a doctor who cared for his patients, whom I would not trust with my own life. A doctor who cares senses his own limitations long before they have been reached. His concern acts as a fail-safe device—a warning system when he needs help. Unwillingness to refer patients to other specialists is a sign of arrogance—not really caring about the well-being of the patient.

One of the really great and good doctors in my community, a general practitioner in his 60s, was recovering from a massive second coronary in our coronary-care unit. He had a huge practice and had not limited his work after his first heart attack thirteen years earlier. This coronary came out of the blue and will ultimately force him to retirement, although that was the furthest thing from his mind when I visited him four days after his attack. He was pale, reasonably comfortable, fully alert, and angrier than depressed over the situation. But he was not taking well to his doctor's recommendation that he retire:

"The bastard thinks I'm ready for the shelf," Peter said. "Who the hell's going to take care of these people?" He waived a small, thick notebook filled with loose pages of patients' names, office appointments, nursing home visits, et cetera. This was Peter's pocket file cabinet—a potpourri of scribbled clinical notes and reminders which he flipped through incessantly as he made his hospital rounds each day. Palm pilot was a gadget totally foreign to this man of the past.

As he thumbed through the book, almost forgetting where he was, his eyes lit upon two or three patients he had recently referred to me for surgery.

"How's that old duffer, Ostrowski? You know, the gall bladder I sent you? Nice people, George, treat 'em well. I remember Ostrowski from way back when he was blinded trying to cross a picket line. Stupid bastard he was."

Then he came upon Mary Jaspers, a sad case with inoperable breast cancer. "Mary still OK? Did you get her home from the hospital yet?" He was still flipping through his portable file cabinet.

"For God's sake, Peter," I interrupted, "will you forget your damned patients and just concentrate on getting over this coronary?"

"The bastard thinks he's going to put me on the shelf. Who the hell's going to pick up this crew of patients?"

Peter knew he was finished but wanted me to agree with him. I hadn't the heart to do otherwise. "You'll be back in a month driving yourself as usual. You're too thickheaded to quit," I said, choking a bit.

He gave me a sidelong glance and said, "You lying bastard."

That was Peter. He cared for his patients and his patients knew it. They said it with dozens of get-well cards—humorous cards that poked fun at the medical profession, the greedy docs, the golf-playing docs, the suave, the polished superspecialists. **They sent these cards to Peter because they knew he cared for them—and because they cared for him.**

Time Out!

Is it possible that a totally incompetent doctor can care very much about his or her patients? And if so, where does that leave the naïve patient, impressed by how much his doctor cares about him only to find out, once a disaster strikes, that the doctor has no real knowledge of disease?

Caring may count but it surely must be considered a minimum requirement of the good physician. And yet the chapter is entitled: The Most Important Sign of a Good Doctor.

The selection process rapidly eliminates the incompetent doctor. Recall that a caring doctor knows when and to what extent he or she must make use of fellow specialists, knows when tests must be ordered and knows when hospitalization is indicated.

A grossly incompetent physician, no matter that he cares, will soon be discovered by his fellow physicians, by hospital nurses, by bizarre laboratory or X-ray requests and so forth. The diagnostic and therapeutic process does not occur in a vacuum. There are too many eyes and ears watching physicians and nurses, and the incompetent doctor, though he cares, soon is discovered and eliminated. His reputation fails and this becomes obvious.

Caring remains the most important sign of a good doctor, but you must be slow to make that judgment and pay attention to all the indicators contained in subsequent chapters of this book.

Look before you keep!

Chapter 8: Time Out for Some Objections

"caring and curing"

Chapter summary: This chapter shows why objective criteria can never be developed to weed out the bad doctors or embellish the reputation of the good doctors. This is not to say that any attempt to regulate good medical practice is useless. But the most brilliant doctor in the world does not necessarily care about his or her patients, and that is what really defines the good doctor. Some objections to my thesis are covered in this chapter. These will all be expanded on in subsequent chapters.

"Now wait just a minute. I'm not interested in whether my doctor cares or not. I'm looking for a well-trained scientific physician, one who knows all the latest innovations in medicine. Don't give me that lonely-hearts jazz. I'm looking for a doctor, not a hand-holding expert."

This objection would have made a lot of sense seventy years ago. There were many poorly trained doctors then. The problem today is precisely the opposite. All doctors are well-trained, but that hasn't eliminated incompetency. That's why recertifying examinations, advocated by consumerists, are not likely to prove much. The vast majority of physicians will pass these exams with flying colors, proving that they have the scientific facts in their heads. But these exams cannot pick out and eliminate crass mercenaries who are in medicine for the buck and nothing else. **Testing will not eliminate irresponsibility, erratic clinical**

behavior, carelessness, poor communication with patients, callousness, or therapeutic adventurism.

What is a good doctor? He is much more than a well-trained technician or a scientist with a head full of facts. The practice of medicine remains more art than science, more humanism than technology. Indeed, there is much to suggest that science and technology have somehow perverted the art of medicine and dehumanized the physician. The decision to apply or misapply that technology is often a judgment of the heart rather than the head. **Caring and curing cannot be separated.** If you are looking for good scientific physicians, they are all around you. Most of them will qualify. But if you are looking for a good physician, start by looking for a human being who cares about people.

A few more objections—there are many more!

"You seem to be antiscientific. Why not return to the old-fashioned G.P. who was long on compassion and short on scientific medicine? He'll hold your hand all the way to the grave and then blame the fates because he couldn't diagnose what any well-trained physician of today could figure out with his eyes closed."

Not at all. No one is advocating an antiscientific position. Modern medicine is producing excellent physicians and I have no desire to return to the ignorance of the past. **But modernism is also breeding a good number of fat cats, physicians with one hand on the pulse and the other on the purse**. Because they really don't care about their patients, they jam their offices full of patients, give but a few minutes to each complaint, fail to tie loose ends together, pass the buck from one specialist to another under the cloak of "double checking", and end up practicing damned poor medicine. Because they don't care, they have absolutely no interest in the human side of medicine—the art of their profession. They communicate very infrequently with families, who are left emotionally distressed because they can't seem to find out what's happening to their loved ones.

The list of defaults by certain members of the medical profession is too long to enumerate here. But scientific knowledge is not one of them. That's precisely why you can search until doomsday to find effective, objective, criteria for choosing a good doctor.

"I don't see how in the world I am going to be able to tell that a doctor cares. He could easily put on a great act for my benefit. Really! The whole thing seems so vague to me."

A physician can easily seem interested when bored, attentive when distracted, and friendly when he'd rather go fishing. We all do that on occasion. But caring for people is a full-time job, and the phonies don't do well at all. In fact, it is far easier for the physician to fake scientific knowledge than to fake caring for people. That's why the charlatan did so well many years ago when people were less informed and there were no certifying committees to check on a doctor's work. The effort and talent required to pull off a full-time fake job of sincerely caring for patients and going that extra mile is just not in the charlatan's makeup. He may fool you for a visit or two but, being aware of what to look for, you'll soon figure him out.

"Faith healers care too. So where does that leave me? I might as well be treated by a cultist."

The point is you're not going to a faith healer. You're going to a licensed physician, preferably one who is certified by his specialty board. That means she's had about eight or nine years of postgraduate education, about double the time it takes to get any other kind of doctorate degree. So you shouldn't be concerned about a doctor's credentials.

At the risk of sounding repetitious, **I must emphasize again that credentials don't guarantee a good doctor**. If they did, this book wouldn't be necessary—all you'd have to do is check your doctor's diplomas and certificates and the problem would evaporate. Credentials are a minimum check on a physician's competency. They say nothing about his sense of responsibility and his willingness to pursue his profession in the fullest, Hippocratic tradition.

I bring these objections up, like clay pigeons, for a purpose. There is a popular misconception about incompetent doctors which underlies legislative and consumer-advocacy plans that try to guarantee high-quality medical care by certifying the competency of physicians. The public recognizes that all doctors are not good, that some are just plain incompetent and unfit to practice medicine. **But they make the fundamental mistake of thinking that these doctors are incompetent because of their lack of knowledge.** So they try to devise laws, rules and regulations with which to check a doctor's scientific knowledge and eliminate him if he falls below a certain level.

These schemes won't work and I hope you see why. Physicians receive an excellent medical education, and their daily contacts with their colleagues keep them up to date in valid, well-tested medical information. The fact that they may not keep up with the latest fad or gimmick is probably a genuine advantage to the public. Genuine medical knowledge just does not change as fast as the news media would lead you to believe. Frontier medicine, the stuff in the headlines, belongs in the medical centers where, under controlled conditions, it is tested and retested and the results, when proven, are passed to the public via the community practitioner.

New medical knowledge is very much like raw material. It must be worked with until the final distillate, a small part of the original investigation, becomes a valid part of the medical practice.

The problem of incompetency is not something testing is going to find and eliminate. Incompetency is a function of a doctor's character, his ethical standards, and his image of himself and his patients. That's why I have insisted that you are a far better judge of a doctor's competency than any certifying agency. Only you can tell if you are being managed in a professionally responsible manner.

Time Out!

See above!

Chapter 9: Finding a Doctor in a New Community

"once upon a time"

Chapter summary: People change living and work locations many times in their lives. They no longer reside in the same neighborhood for generations. They therefore change primary care doctors very frequently, and this can be disconcerting, if not dangerous. This chapter tells you some of the basic things you need to do before you leave for a new community. Don't just pick up your belongings and leave town. Pay a last visit to your present doctor, gather your records, ask her if she can give you a list of all the board-certified primary care doctors in your new community. Plan ahead is the message of this chapter. It may save you grief; it may save your life.

Once upon a time, as every fairy tale starts, people lived in close-knit neighborhoods. Each community had its church, school, and corner drugstore, each within a stone's throw of the other, and people socialized in an intimate, communal life. **Patients and physicians established lifelong relationships which often were as social, religious or political as they were medical**.

My father was a general practitioner, and I recall some of these relationships vividly. Sunday morning church services, the local softball league for fathers and sons, Saturday evening cookouts, fireworks displays—these and similar events brought all the citizens together on an equal footing where informality was the rule rather that the exception. The system was stable and the neighborhood physician was chosen as a family physician simply because he was there. There was no need to think about your choice. And a rather simple process it was, because you knew your doctor rather well.

Mobility has changed all that and destroyed the intimacy of communal neighborhood living. Indeed, mobility is one of the radical changes in our lifestyle which has made it difficult to achieve a satisfactory relationship with a doctor. The birth, life, illnesses and death of a person were once within the panoramic vision of a single family doctor, but this is rarely true today. These existential experiences are likely to take place far apart, as people move from one place to another, seven to ten times in a lifetime. **You will never know the physician who attended you at birth and probably won't be able to recall the physicians who delivered your children.** A kaleidoscope of physicians will care for you through your inevitable illnesses and yet, again, a new personality and strange face will minister to you when you are dying.

These are the facts of mobile suburban life which cannot be wished away. Unlike the happy ending to every fairy tale, you are not destined to live happily forevermore, but must face your existence, mold it when you can, and make the best of it. Planning ahead for the best medical care you can get and the best physicians you can find is a very important part of your life and starts the moment you find yourself without a personal doctor.

Let's assume that you have just moved to a new town and do not have a physician. What happens to your medical records when you change locations? If you're fortunate enough to have a doctor you can trust, you will do two things before leaving for your new residence:

First: Ask your doctor to recommend two or three board-certified, primary-care physicians in your new community. She has a national directory of all physicians, which include their ages, addresses and specialty training. Ask her what type of physician she recommends for you and your family based on her knowledge of your specific needs. This will be a good start, although it is not absolutely necessary if circumstances don't permit it.

Second: Ask your doctor to give you a copy of all your medical records and those of your family. This should include information from her office files as well as any available hospital records. They may include the following vital information about you: (1) organs removed and findings at the time of surgery; (2) X-ray and scan reports; (3) laboratory findings; (4) comments and judgments about your health by your doctor; (5) response to drugs, including allergies and idiosyncrasies.

If your physician does not wish to make these records available to you, have a frank discussion with her and seek legal counsel if she remains adamant. The law is not yet clear, but these records are probably your legal property. Most physicians recognize this right and will more than cooperate with you in this request. **Under no circumstances should you change residence several times in a lifetime, generating medical records on yourself here and there and not have them together and readily available for each subsequent doctor treating you**. It makes no sense to have your record start over each time you move. Biologically speaking, you are still the same person you were; your medical record will be of great value to a new physician.

So now you've settled down in your new home, met the neighbors, and found the supermarket. When do you start searching for a family doctor? Most people wait until they're sick and wonder why it's so hard to get an appointment or find a doctor. They end up in an emergency room because they are crisis-oriented about illness, seeking advice only when seriously ill and paying no attention to preventive examinations.

Plan Ahead. Start your search for a good doctor while you're feeling well and have time to make a careful choice. Many factors have to be taken into consideration. A family with young children will need an internist (or family practitioner) and a pediatrician. Both will act as primary-care physicians. You and your spouse may wish separate primary physicians. Ideally, a single doctor should take care of both of you, but this doesn't always work out because of personality differences. It's a good idea to discuss this issue together before making a choice. One physician who serves an entire family is far less expensive than several doctors. Somehow she knows something about your pocketbook and your medical expenses and will tend to go easy when she has the loyalty of an entire family. Since the interrelationships within a family are much better understood by a family doctor, this may give your physician important insights into individual stresses within the family.

Doctors are busy people. Be prepared to wait several weeks for that first appointment. Since you've planned ahead, this won't matter. When making this appointment, emphasize to the receptionist that you would like to schedule enough time for a complete, routine physical examination. This may take forty-five minutes, depending on a number of variables. Most conscientious physicians usually allow that much time for new patients, so you shouldn't have much trouble making such an arrangement.

Should you get any jazz, such as, "doctor is very busy and only allows ten minutes per visit"—or anything like that—start running! You've already found a dud. Look again! Roughly translated, the receptionist is saying: "Look, buddy, my boss is in the business of making a lot of money by running patients through as quickly as possible. She's looking for major medical problems only and building a huge clientele for big income. I'm busy too, so don't look for much sympathy from me."

A good doctor must be thorough and know everything she can about you, your family, your work, your lifestyle. This isn't possible if her practice has outgrown the time she has available for you. You may even have to pay more for the luxury of a doctor's time, since the low volume physician is faced with the same fixed expenses as her busier competitor. But if you have to choose between an inexpensive assembly-line doctor and a real professional who spends plenty of time with you, choose the latter.

Time Out!

The idea that your doctor will search out a new doctor for you in a different part of the country (or world!!) is rather far-fetched. I suppose it can be done if you know him or her very well and you push hard enough. The odds are she will tell you she knows no doctors in East Blah Blah and you're on your own again.

At least be sure to get your records. That is a minimum and you should push very hard if you run into any resistance.

Chapter 10: A Good Doctor Works Hard

"pulling a rabbit out of a hat"

Chapter Summary: How do you evaluate your new-found physician? This chapter begins the process of showing you. It boils down to how hard he works at evaluating your health or diagnosing your illness. The whole point of this chapter is that diagnosis is not some kind of magic rabbit-out-of-a-hat syndrome. It takes very hard and detailed work. You will want to refer to this chapter before going to see your doctor. It will help you judge whether he lives up to the thoroughness required of a good diagnostician.

Star Trek, a space travel television series many years ago, featured a physician called "Bones." He used 22nd century diagnostic technology to figure out what ailed his spaceship mates. The patient was placed under a probing shield, lights flashed on a large screen and the diagnosis came out on a computer printout within microseconds.

Many people have the notion that clinical diagnosis is just that uncanny. The whole thing has something of the aura of a mystery about it. We physicians are given far more credit for our detective powers than we deserve. Diagnosis is not an easy thing and does not lend itself to simple formulas or magic incantations sprinkled with alchemy. **A good doctor works hard at making a diagnosis**. You don't have to have a Ph.D. in medicine to sense his thoroughness or its absence. How hard he works at his diagnoses is an important criterion in judging how good your doctor really is.

Let's see how this principle applies. Evaluating a new patient is going to take about forty-five minutes to an hour, depending on the complexity of the problem and the pace of the physician. If you have made an appointment for a complete physical examination by your new doctor (as I suggested earlier), your job is to check him out while he is checking you. **Get it?** While he's evaluating your health, you're evaluating his competency. We've already talked about the doctor who cares; now let's concentrate on how hard he works for you.

Evaluating the general health of a patient begins with a thorough history. This is a precise interrogation and may take fifteen to twenty minutes. The doctor may do this part of the examination as you sit opposite him (the preferable way) or while he is examining you. **An accurate and thorough history is the most important part of the diagnostic process, far more significant than any laboratory, X-ray or other special test which your doctor may order.**

The history will include the following important areas:

1. **The chief complaint and present illness**: This is a statement of your present medical problem as you see it. If you have come for a routine examination you may not have any specific complaints, in which case your doctor will go on to the other parts of the history listed below. But if you do have a complaint, your physician must concentrate on this symptom and try to draw important clues about your illness by questioning you in depth about it. Symptoms don't come in organized, textbook patterns and it is the rare patient who can discuss his or her symptoms in a scientific way. After all, if you have had no previous experience with the symptoms of disease, you aren't expected to be able to write a textbook about it. That is your doctor's job. He must spend as much time as it takes to refine your symptoms into a pattern to define the nature of the disease process.

Taking a good history is like doing a good piece of detective work. Your doctor has to search for clues. Sometimes the diagnosis is fairly clear-cut by the end of the first interview. At other times, your doctor may have to go over the same ground several times before he picks up the path that leads to a diagnosis.

The issue is complicated by the fact that the body may reflect symptoms in one area when the problem is in an entirely different spot. Other times, though the body accurately reports the true cause of the problem, the patient is unable to express himself because of vagueness of the symptoms. Sometimes the mind exaggerates or minimizes certain symptoms for a variety of psychological reasons. The doctor sifts out these nuances as he becomes familiar with his patient's personality.

Complicating all this is the occasional problem of sifting out the real symptom from a set of apparent symptoms used by the patient to gain admission in the doctor's office. I call this game the **"ticket of admission,"** a ploy used by some patients who feel their doctor will not pay attention if they come out immediately with the real reason for their visit. This may not be a conscious process.

The mysteries of human behavior are not the subject of this book. I shall not attempt to discuss the secondary motivations which drive patients to doctors, the curious games which go on between doctors and their patients, the subtleties of the human body reporting abnormalities, the difficulties of the human consciousness in integrating these complaints, the confusion and, on occasion, deviousness of the human speech in reporting them and, finally, the frailties of a doctor's observations and judgments in putting it all together. Medicine is sometimes called an art form and the taking of a proper and accurate history is a creative and imaginative process. **All subsequent examinations and special tests depend ultimately on the thoroughness and accuracy of the history; hence its paramount importance in the diagnostic process.**

Your chief complaint is the takeoff point for the entire interview. Let us assume that your problem is chest pain and that you have been suffering with it for about three weeks. A good physician will spend a great deal of time going over this pain with you in some detail.

He will want to know about the nature of the pain, whether it is knife-like or dull or more of a pressure sensation; whether it is severe or only moderately discomforting; where it is located in your chest; whether the pain radiates somewhere else or merely stays in one place; whether it is steady or comes and goes; whether it is relieved or worsened by lying down; whether it is associated with other symptoms such as shortness of breath, nausea, or vomiting; whether you have ever had this pain in the past and, if so, when, under what conditions and so on. He will want to know if you strained yourself before this pain started; whether other symptoms preceded the development of the pain; and so on.

While all of this is going on, an astute physician will be sizing up your answers, trying to decide how accurate you are in reporting symptoms, whether you tend to play up or play down pains and discomforts, whether there are any subconscious factors at work distorting the symptoms as you feel them or as you report them. If this is your first visit with the particular doctor, he will be very careful about how much weight he gives your story and description of your symptoms until he knows and understands you better. That is why it is crucial to have a primary physician, to get to know him, to let him get to know you. **Patients who change doctors frequently, use emergency rooms, or go to doctors only when in severe distress, simply do not understand the subtle nature of the diagnostic process and how important is the familiarity between a doctor and his patient.**

2. **Family History**: Since many illnesses are inherited, a good medical history attempts to uncover problems in your family that may have a bearing on your health. Some serious illnesses most apt to have an inheritable basis are: cancer; cardiovascular disease; diabetes; chronic infections such as tuberculosis; kidney disease; congenital defects. There are others but it serves no useful purpose to enumerate them here. The important point is that an adequate evaluation of your present health requires detailed information about your family history. Knowing this, **you should prepare yourself for the interview by finding out as much as you can about your family medical history**.

3. **Past history**: We don't live in a biological vacuum. Your current health is largely a manifestation of all your past illnesses, which your physician must ascertain before he can make any rational decision about your present status. **This is why your previous records are so valuable.** They include significant birth and development problems, childhood illnesses, major operations, and any condition that required hospitalization. When you give these records to your new doctor, observe whether he refers to them. This will give you a clue about how thorough he is.

4. **Drug History**: Your doctor should request a complete rundown on drugs you have used, their purpose and whether you ever had any adverse reactions. Drug reactions are a serious cause

of death and disability in this country and are far commoner than patients realize or doctors like to admit. A conscientious doctor spends a great deal of time going over each drug a patient has used in the past.

5. **Social history**: This includes a review of your work and social habits; whether you smoke and, if so, what and how much; how much alcohol you consume; what types of food you enjoy and whether your nutritional habits are disease prone; what type of work you do and any signs of occupational hazards connected with your work; marital status, with emphasis on signs of domestic stress, and so on.

6. **Review of systems**: The body is divided into ten organs systems:

- Skin
- Special senses: vision, hearing, smell
- Cardio-pulmonary system
- Genito-urinary system
- Gastro-intestinal system
- Nervous system
- Musculo-skeletal system
- Endocrine system
- Blood-forming system
- Immunologic system

Each of these systems, when failing, produces characteristic symptoms and your doctor should review them in an orderly fashion, trying to uncover early symptoms of disease. This part of the history may take a few minutes or could go on for twenty to thirty minutes. Subtle symptoms in any one of these body systems will require more detailed questions and may lead to a variety of tests designed to ferret out early disease.

A good history is absolutely essential for a proper evaluation of your health status. You can undergo $1000 worth of fancy X-rays, scans and blood tests but, without a proper history, the exams are of very little value. The ability of a physician to predict serious disease based on your living style, for example, is wrapped up in a carefully taken social history. The patient who thinks the $500 "executive" physical examination, consisting of a string of X-rays and some blood tests, is a guarantee of good health is dangerously deceived. Tests are only valuable if they follow a thorough sifting of a patient's history. They mean very little unless they happen to uncover some disease not causing any symptoms whatsoever.

After he has taken your history, your doctor should ask you to step into his examining room for a physical examination. This can only be done with you completely undressed. The doctor who fumbles through sweaters and shirts with his stethoscope is not doing it to save you embarrassment. He's trying to cut corners. You should find a new doctor. **A good doctor works hard at it. Always keep this principle in mind. Watch your doctor carefully**.

There is no mystery to the physical examination. After you've had such an examination with your new physician, review this chapter and see how many of the following he actually carried out on you. It is an excellent test of his thoroughness—of how hard he works at taking care of you.

The vital signs: (There are four.)

- Blood pressure: Preferably taken in both arms for comparison
- Pulse: Usually measured at the wrist and timed with a wristwatch
- Respiration: The number of respirations per minute, also counted with a wristwatch.
- Temperature: Taken orally or rectally.

Skin:

A thorough check of your skin for precancerous moles, dermatitis, jaundice, pallor, and so on; skin cancer often affects the parts of the body exposed to sun (face, forehead, nape of neck, ears, nose, backs of hands), so particular attention is paid to these areas.

Head:

Shape and scalp infections

Eyes:

Vision may be tested, although I do not personally think this is a necessary part of a thorough examination in a healthy-appearing adult.

- Intra-ocular pressure: A test for glaucoma done by using eye drops to anesthetize the eye, then placing a small pressure gauge against the eyeball for a reading. It can also be done with more sophisticated devices.
- The inside of the eye, or fundus, may reflect early hypertension and various stages of diabetes. It is examined with an ophthalmoscope in a semi-darkened room. It is a very important part of a general exam.

Ears:

The drums are examined with an otoscope. Hearing may be grossly tested with a wristwatch held close to the ears. This really is inexact but most physicians are not equipped or trained to carry out audiometric exams.

Nose, throat, mouth:

Usually checked with a tongue depressor and flashlight; a small angled mirror is used to look down your throat at the vocal cords, to look especially for early throat cancer.

Neck:

The thyroid gland, major arteries to the brain, major veins to the heart and lymph nodes are all carefully examined by feeling various parts of the neck and listening to the neck arteries.

Chest:

Using the stethoscope, the physician listens to your heart and lungs. He often thumps your chest, using one finger as a hammer against another to detect fluid in the chest or something causing consolidation in your lungs.

Breasts:

A careful examination of the female breast for breast cancer, cysts, and other tumors is carried out. The examination also includes the axillae (arm pits) and the depressions just above the collarbones on both sides.

Abdomen:

He feels your abdomen for lumps or enlarged organs and listens to it with his stethoscope. The examination also includes the groins for hernias and other lumps.

Genitals:

An examination of the testicles in males and an internal examination of the womb and ovaries in females.

Rectum:

Done with the finger to check for tumors, hemorrhoids and, in the male, an enlarged prostrate gland.

Extremities:

The reflexes are checked; pulses are checked in the groins, behind each knee, and at the ankles.

Back:

He gently punches over your kidneys located in each flank, trying to elicit any tenderness; the shape and alignment of the spine is also checked.

Well there you have it. I've avoided some of the more detailed parts of the examination because they're a bit subtle and something you're not likely to see your doctor do. But there are other aspects that you should be especially alert to. There are several key parts to a physical examination which, because they are time consuming, the less-than-adequate doctor tends to avoid. This is cutting corners and is completely unacceptable.

If the following examinations were not done, you have not undergone a complete physical examination:

- Blood pressure measurement; preferably in two arms.
- Examination of the inside of your eye, the so-called funduscopic examination; this must be done in a semi darkened room with an ophthalmoscope.
- Breast examination; pelvic examination; Pap smear for all adult females.
- Rectal examination

I am not suggesting that the rest of the physical examination is less necessary. But these four are the time consumers, the inconvenient parts of the examination for the doctor and the ones most likely to be avoided by the incompetent physician. They are bellboys for you, channel markers of an adequate physical examination. If you have not had them, the examination is not complete and serious problems may be left undetected. Remember, a good doctor works hard at it. These last four examinations are your way of examining your new doctor.

I recall being asked to examine a thirty-five year old male who had been treated by his physician for nine months for persistent diarrhea. Failing to stop the diarrhea with a number of drugs, he sent the man to me for my opinion. I did a rectal examination and discovered a cancer the size of my fist. It was so obvious that a chimpanzee could have made the diagnosis. I asked the patient if his physician had performed the examination. He told me that it had not been done in over six visits to his doctor for diarrhea. This is criminal neglect. Why did it happen? Because the doctor has gotten into the habit of avoiding rectal examinations. He had practiced this way for so many years that this simple diagnostic test, which takes two minutes to do, completely escaped his habit of thinking and he went on treating the diarrhea for nine months without a diagnosis. Does he know a rectal exam ought to be done? Of course he does!

Needless to say, each subsequent visit with your doctor for the same illness will not involve an entire history and examination. Follow-up examinations, depending on the progress you are making, may require just a few minutes to check how things are going, readjust your drug dosage, and be certain no new problems are developing. Likewise, an urgent or acute disease may militate against such a thorough interview and examination. As soon as the emergency is over, however, a complete examination should be carried out.

Another exception is when either you or your doctor is not in the right frame of mind for a complete examination. It is proper, under these circumstances, to defer the examination to a more appropriate time. For example, I recently examined a woman with a lump in her breast. She was so emotionally distraught that she could barely keep her mind on my questions. The anguish in her facial expressions, the wringing of her hands, the inattention to my questions, all signaled that this was not the time to explore the details of her family and past history. My mandate here was to be brief, sympathetic and reassuring. This is the art of medicine. The long interview and complete examination had to wait another day. I told her I believed the lump was an innocent cyst filled with fluid, and removed the fluid in one minute with a needle. She could feel for herself that the lump had disappeared. I scheduled her for a breast X-ray and told her to come back in a week. When the breast X-ray revealed no suspicious problem and the lump had not recurred, I told her to return in one month so I could reevaluate the area and do a complete examination.

Doctors become fatigued like anyone else, often finding themselves at the end of a long day or week unable to concentrate on any new problems, and yet still faced with three or four new patients who require complete examinations. Under these circumstances, it is in the best interest of both doctor and patient to defer the examination. A simple explanation to a patient is usually sufficient, providing the examination is carried out at a later date.

With these few exceptions, anything less than a thorough examination such as I have described is a sign that something is wrong. Beware of the doctor who listens briefly to your chief complaint, asks very few questions, performs a rather cursory examination of the area of your complaint, prescribes a simple medication, pats you on the shoulder, reassures you and tells you to come back in a week. **You've wasted your time and your money and risked your health.**

Time Out!

A doctor spending 45 minutes doing a medical exam? Come off it. The last time a doctor spent 45 minutes watching anything was the third quarter of a tight football game.

Is this all realistic? I ask patients to watch the doctor carefully for a **twist of his wrist**—when he not-so-subtly looks at his watch to be sure he is staying within the 7-10 minutes allowed by his HMO.

So how do you get around this handcuffing of doctors by HMOs? It is easy. Just remember that he must see patients **on an average of every 7-10 minutes** or some such low, magical number set by the system. If you are demanding enough time with him or her, he will rapidly adjust and spend whatever time it takes to keep you happy and then make up for it with other patients. **As usual, the squeaky axle gets the grease.**

Chapter 11: The Word "Doctor" Means Teacher

"I have a question, teacher"

Chapter summary: This is the key chapter of this book. The whole essence of the doctor-patient relationship rests on the skill, enthusiasm and thoroughness of the doctor's instincts as a good teacher for his or her patients. It does very little good if the only thing she does is manage the immediate problem for which you went to her. What is critical is that she begins the process of teaching you about your illnesses, the risk factors endangering your well-being and how you can change your lifestyle for the better. This is teaching, and it is of the essence of good doctoring. The chapter attempts to spell this out in some detail. Teaching is a time-consuming process and not something that can be rushed in a five-minute visit to the doctor. If you do not feel that you are in the presence of an inspiring teacher when you visit your doctor, I strongly advise you to begin looking around again.

I once asked a group of interns what they thought the practice of medicine was all about. The answers varied, of course, but none really hit the mark. Most of them emphasized the diagnosis and treatment of disease. I could not quarrel with this answer. Certainly that's what we do, but for what purpose? What are we trying to accomplish?

The word "doctor" means teacher, and it is the doctor's responsibility to teach her patients the art of healthy living.

Those patients who are in excellent health must be taught to preserve it. Those who have an ailment, whether acute or chronic, must be taught how to restore and maintain their health in the best possible state under the circumstances.

Many years ago a colleague of mine was looking around for a place to practice. He initially decided on a large medical group on the West coast and went there to be interviewed by the administrator and to tour the facility.

The outpatient department was a huge operation which treated several thousand patients a year. While walking through the department, the administrator informed my colleague that he was permitted ten minutes with each patient.

"Ten minutes!" the doctor said. "But how will I have time to teach?"

"Oh, we don't have medical students here," the administrator hastened to point out.

He had missed the point of the question. My colleague, a fine and conscientious physician, understood at the onset of his career that teaching is of the essence of the doctor-patient relationship. **His patients are his students.**

A patient comes to a physician because she wishes to find out what ails her, what she must do to get well, what the outcome of her illness will be, and what she must do to preserve her health in the future. While it is true that she also wishes to be cured or made more comfortable, the patient instinctively realizes that a good part of the treatment depends on her intelligent application of good health measures that should be spelled out for her by her physician. That is why the patient asks questions. She is a student and wishes to know the cause of an ailment and how to remain healthy in the future.

Once the doctor has completed your examination, the most important part of the visit takes place. You return to her consulting room for a thorough discussion of your health and recommendations for future care.

How good a "teacher" is your doctor?

This is a vital checkpoint for your evaluation—a chance to check out your new physician as a teacher. Here are some questions to keep in mind. Refer to them before and immediately after your visit and see how well he scores:

1. **How well does your doctor communicate with you?** A good teacher communicates with her student. Is she talking to you, above you or below you? Is she trying to impress you with the jargon of her trade? Anyone can do that, but it's not good teaching and often is a sign of some inferiority complex to boot.

2. **Do you feel at ease talking with her?** Teaching is communicating and this is a two-way street. Does she seem accessible or removed? Does she answer your questions directly and forthrightly, or with a series of evasions and pompous put-downs? She can be the most informed, scientific physician in the world, but it does you no good if she can't get what's in her skull inside your skull and receive, evaluate and respond to your questions in plain, crisp language.

3. **What ought she to teach you?**

a. The present state of your health: if excellent, how do you maintain it? If you have a problem, what is it or what tests have to be done to figure it out? How complex are these tests, what are their risks, costs, and inconveniences? How uncomfortable are they? What are your experiences with them likely to be?

b. Your present living style and its relationship to your health. What are you doing that is likely to impair your health? What ought you do to improve or maintain your health? Does she sense anything that bodes ill for the future? In other words, what risk factors does she perceive in the way you are doing things? What good does it do to discover that you have a high cholesterol level or high blood pressure and not admonish you about the horribly high cholesterol foods you eat, the two packs of cigarettes you consume daily, and the excess caloric baggage you're carrying around in your midsection?

c. Drugs and their hazards. I cannot emphasize this area enough. In the past, we have greatly underestimated the amount of disability and death caused by prescription drugs. Let me take just one example. Digitalis is an effective heart stimulant. Used intelligently, it can save your life when you are suffering from heart failure. Certain illnesses require long-term use of this drug. It is also a very dangerous drug. To make matters worse, it is extremely incompatible with a number of drugs readily available in any drug store without a prescription. Whenever a physician places a patient on Digitalis she must go over the ground rules carefully for the safe use of this drug. This takes time, effort and good communication. Failure to do this may result in your death. Other drugs are equally dangerous. The warning symptoms of a toxic reaction to each drug must be explained in detail to you. Here the enthusiastic teacher becomes the good doctor and a failure to teach becomes gross incompetence.

There is almost no correlation between a doctor's scientific knowledge and her ability to teach her patient about the hazards of drugs. Very little effort is spent in medical school to teach doctors the art of communicating information to their patients. The whole education of a physician is premised on a misconception of her role. She is looked upon as a professional trained to figure out what is wrong with people and how to correct the problem. That is why the modern physician does such a good job treating acute critical illness and such a bad job educating people about their health habits and living styles. When the illness is acute and susceptible to the application of scientific principles and technological devices, where all that is needed from the patient is acceptance, the "fix-it" training of the physician comes through and she does an excellent job.

But this is such a small part of a doctor's world. Most of his time is spent with relatively healthy patients who are seeking reassurance and relief, or with patients suffering chronic disease who need, besides relief of their symptoms, education about their problems, friendship and caring, adjustments of their lifestyles, and so on. **In all of these areas, a deficiency in the education and orientation of the modern physician prevents her from serving as a health teacher**. Those physicians who have been able to overcome this deficiency make far better doctors because they are fulfilling their "teaching role" over and above their "fix-it" role.

One of the chief difficulties with today's overspecialized health system is that very few physicians know enough about their patients' living styles to be able to educate them for a healthier life. The specialist defines her role along her specialty line, when often the cause of the breakdown in the organ she is called on to treat is removed from her area of expertise. The role of stress in the development of hypertension is a case in point. Hypertension often leads to disabling illness such as strokes, and yet the neurologist, expert in the diagnosis and treatment of strokes, knows little to nothing about the stresses occurring in each of her patients that may have caused the hypertension and the stroke in the first place. A good physician comes to understand this and can prevent catastrophes by frequent, thorough discussions about stress and living habits with his patients.

The critical question you must ask yourself:

The most highly trained doctor can be useless if she doesn't cover the big picture by teaching her patient about good health and how to maintain it. **The single most important question you must ask yourself after talking to your new doctor is this: How well do I understand my body, its illnesses, the drugs I am to take and the regimen I must follow to keep my health or restore it?**

If your answer is less than enthusiastic, if you feel rather empty after this appointment, if you're walking out with a prescription in hand, an appointment for a blood test and another appointment with this doctor, and you know next to nothing about what I've been talking about, you've made a bad choice of doctors and you'd better go back to "go" and start all over again.

A case in point:

Let's see if we can make the whole thing more concrete. Let's take your chief complaint—in this case, recurring and severe headaches—and illustrate the difference between a good doctor and one who isn't worth the time of day.

We'll do this by sending you to both with the same problem. We'll assume that you've never been to either in your life.

You are a forty-two year-old woman, a homemaker, with two teenaged children. You belong to a few civic-action committees and play some tennis. You have some free time on your hands as your responsibilities at home diminish. If you're a male or your situation differs, just change the description. The same principles apply.

Your immediate problem is a severe and recurring headache, something you haven't experienced in the past, and something causing you real concern. Your eyeglasses are fine; the problem is not eyestrain. You've tried a few home remedies with no lasting relief.

With very little thought as to what type of doctor you should see, you choose Dr. Smith, a local internist, whose name you got from your tennis friends. Your experience with Dr. Smith was not satisfying and she certainly didn't solve your problem. She seemed over-busy and harassed. She spent two rushed minutes listening to your complaint, took your blood pressure, mumbled something about it being okay and told you the headaches were either tension or migraine. It was somewhat of a mystery to you how she arrived at her diagnosis, considering she spent so little time and did little more than examine your eyes and check your blood pressure. She prescribed a medicine for the migraine and something to "relax your nerves" but told you nothing about the pills and gave you no further instructions about returning for another visit.

The headaches didn't go away. The medicine seemed to alleviate matters for a short period, or maybe you just decided not to be bothered for a while.

A few days passed, the headaches were no better and you began to look around again. Perhaps this time you did some checking before seeing another doctor. You found out that Dr. Jones enjoyed a **widespread excellent reputation**.

You were almost overwhelmed by her thorough interview and examination. But what impressed you most was the discussion in her consulting room after the examination. She informed you that the headaches did not appear serious; that they may indeed have been some variant of migraine. Nevertheless, certain aspects of these headaches so disturbed her that she recommended a consultation with a neurologist, one whom she thoroughly endorsed.

But that is not all. She also discovered several important things about your current lifestyle that were far more significant than your headaches:

a. You were smoking too many cigarettes and had already developed wheezes in your lungs, so-called smoker's bronchitis, a forerunner of emphysema. If you stopped smoking you could avoid a catastrophe in the next decade of your life.

b. Though you may hotly deny it, the amount of alcohol that you were consuming both at home and at the tennis court was a telltale sign of future problems. Indeed, she found your liver slightly enlarged, and recommended that some liver tests be done.

c. You weighed about 30 pounds more than your age, height, and skeletal structure required. Moreover, your eating habits had deteriorated over the years— you were inclined toward high-cholesterol foods. Since these may lead to heart disease, she recommended a few blood tests to see if your cholesterol was out of whack. Your family history suggested that early heart disease was a familial problem and this, combined with the excess cigarette consumption, might prove fatal.

d. Finally, she discovered a small groin hernia, which was totally unknown to you, and recommended a surgeon's opinion to see if it should be repaired.

Topping off all this, Dr. Jones agreed to make arrangements with a neurologist for your headaches, a surgeon for your hernia, and the laboratory for the examination of your liver. Because of the wheezes in your lungs, she also recommended a lung scan to be certain you hadn't developed anything more serious, such as lung cancer, and gave you an appointment to return after your consultations and tests.

Without embarrassing you, she pointed out that your habits represented a serious threat to your health and strongly recommended that you give the entire matter some thought before your next visit. You left with the impression that she was thorough and cared about the state of your health without appearing to be a moralist. You pretty much knew that she was right but her reinforcement, particularly from a person who spent her life evaluating health problems, was a very important learning experience. Doing something about it, of course, was up to you.

It doesn't take long to figure out the difference between Drs. Smith and Jones or to realize how important the educational process is in the art of medicine. Neither of these experiences had much to do with the doctors' level of scientific medical knowledge. Chances are if you tested them with written examinations, one would "know" as much as the other. Yet, is there any doubt in your mind which physician is the better doctor?

Time Out!

Enter HMOs, managed care and the gatekeeper lock out

Sir William Osler, a famous medical educator from Johns Hopkins University, once said that the three A's of good doctoring were **Availability, Affability and Ability** and that the first was far the most important. Unless a doctor be available to his or her patients, ability does not matter at all.

In order to save money, managed care systems attempt to limit the availability of physicians in many overt and subtle ways, the most common being to limit the amount of time a doctor spends with patients. This frequently comes down to seven to ten minutes, hardly enough time to be a good teacher of health care.

How can you approach this problem and manage your care while HMOs are attempting at times to mismanage that care?

Eye-wrist contacts:

First, become aware that times have surely changed and your time with the doctor will be severely restricted. You can get a clue about the time rationing with your doctor by watching her eye-wrist contacts. She is checking her watch every minute to be sure she doesn't violate the seven-to-ten minute rule. **If she is looking at a wall behind you, chances are there is a large wall clock for her to watch!**

The time-conscious doctor does not even permit you to dress and go to her consulting room for the teaching part of the relationship. She tells you about your health while you are partially undressed, lying under a white sheet in her examining room, hardly the position for being an intelligent student. Indeed, if you look around you will likely find that the modern doctor's office does not even have a consulting room. All the rooms are devoted to examinations and testing except a little nook she has where she goes to make notes and phone calls.

Once you have noted the rationing of care and the lack of any teaching by your physician, it is time to complain and you must be firm though polite.

Prudent complaining:

Let me make some suggestions about how to go about complaining and getting the biggest bang for your buck. It is probably not a good idea to complain about how bad a teacher your doctor is on the first visit. Swallow hard and go home. Give it some thought. Talk to a friend or two about your experience. Exactly what went wrong with this from your point of view? Did you learn about your present illness? Did she prescribe drugs and talk about the dangers of these drugs? Did she recommend any lab or X-ray tests? Did she explain why she wanted these tests? Did she suggest another kind of specialist and, if so, did she explain why?

Write all this down. Give it some further thought. Write down some challenging questions. Then return for your second visit with this doctor.

Again be a "patient" patient. Let her examine you and discuss things in the brief time allotted by her HMO or your insurance carrier. Ask her the questions you have written down. Do not be ashamed to take out the paper containing these questions. Indeed this is always a good tactic as it shows the doctor that you have given it all some thought and you are serious about the questions. You may find that little piece of paper with the questions on it works magic.

Perhaps it is time to leave this doctor.

If you are still not satisfied (and you have a right to be very demanding)—your health and possibly your life may depend on it—it is time for more serious action. If the doctor works alone you have to talk this over either with her or her office manager. If she is part of a large physician group, bound by insurance rules which attempt to ration health care, you will have to discuss this with some administrator of the program. If aggressive confrontation is simply not a part of your personality, then it is time to leave this doctor and find another either within this group or perhaps with a new doctor in another group.

Chapter 12: Thirteen Dis-eases That Can Kill You.

"an undertaker's dozen"

Chapter Summary: Based on what I have observed over 30 years' of medical practice and in discussing these issues at well over 500 monthly mortality and morbidity conferences with fellow physicians, the thirteen things listed here arise as the most serious problems that can spell a lethal outcome for you, the patient. I list and describe them briefly. In one respect they all seem so self-evident. It is a wonder they ever happen. But they do and they are not a failure so much of a doctor's intelligence, rather they result from too little time with a patient, poor communication, the handcuffing of the doctor by insurance number crunchers and all the other issues talked about in this book. **Read these lethal practices each and every time you pay a visit to your doctor** and do not be afraid to ask questions about them whenever you have any doubts. **This could save your life.**

I've given you some positive indicators of a good doctor. Now, let's look at an incompetent doctor and some of the bad habits that are ingrained in his daily practice. I emphasize again that these faults are not due to a poor education or a lack of scientific knowledge. They are caused by laziness, callousness, greed and similar character deficiencies. They cannot be discovered by certifying examinations or licensing boards, but you can pick them up simply by following the general principles established in this book, and by observing your doctor's behavior closely.

Each of the following thirteen bad habits can be lethal. Most of them are easy to detect if you look for them and ask a few pertinent questions. Let's take them one at a time—be sure you review them before and after each visit to your doctor.

1. Treating symptoms, not diseases

I am sure you know that pain is a symptom of some underlying disease. It just doesn't happen without a reason. You also know that painkillers do not remove the cause of the pain. Relieving the pain without looking for its cause creates a potentially dangerous situation. That's why the instructions on the aspirin bottle warn: "If pain persists, see your doctor."

Most of the aches, pains and feelings of illness that affect you are symptoms of an underlying derangement called a disease. The disease may be simple and short-lived. If detected early, it is easily cured or at least controlled to the point of minimizing damage. Some illnesses, which we call latent, cause no symptoms for a long time. Left undetected, they can cause serious damage without your being even slightly aware of their existence. Cancer, in all its horrible species, is a perfect example.

Under no circumstances should a physician persevere in treating symptoms without a thorough search for the underlying disease. To do so is a completely irresponsible act and leaves you no better off than if you had sought relief by purchasing a nonprescription drug. In fact you're worse off. At least when you tried your own treatment, instinct told you not to persevere beyond a certain point.

That's why you finally decided to see a doctor. By treating symptoms only, your doctor is putting his seal of approval on your illness. He's telling you the symptoms mean nothing serious and will go away with the prescription he has given you.

He is also compounding the problem because the drugs he uses are usually more potent than those you can get on your own, and these can cause their own problems. You could end up worse off with an incompetent doctor than if you had continued treating yourself!

You can easily figure out if your physician is treating symptoms only. Just bear in mind some of the principles you have learned already, especially: **Good doctors are good teachers. A good doctor works hard.**

Let's take an example. Suppose you visit your doctor because you have had diarrhea for four weeks. The cause may be simple and innocuous, such as an irritable bowel. But the diarrhea could also be a warning sign of cancer or a serious form of colitis. An incompetent physician is liable to give you an incomplete examination, rush you through an abbreviated history and prescribe a medication to stop the diarrhea. Or, at best, he may get one X-ray of your intestine, find that it's normal, and then give you a simple medication to eliminate the symptoms.

A good doctor works hard. **Diagnosis almost never comes easy**. It takes time, effort, and perseverance. A good doctor will question you at length about the diarrhea. When did it start? Is it getting worse? How many bowel movements a day? Do they contain blood or mucous? Have your bowel movements been at all formed or are they loose and watery? Any abdominal cramps associated with the diarrhea? Any other associated symptoms? Any weight loss? Have you ever had similar symptoms in the past? Any colitis or intestinal cancer in your family? And on and on.

This line of questioning may take fifteen minutes or so and may be repeated during subsequent visits, differing in details as more information becomes available.

Next, your doctor will carry out a thorough physical examination emphasizing, but not limited to, the digestive system.

At the end of the interview and examination, a good doctor will sit with you and explain his thought process. This is the teaching part of good medicine. He may not have arrived at a diagnosis. But he has some ideas, some clues that he must follow. He may give you a list of possible explanations for your diarrhea. This approach, called **the differential diagnosis**, leads to certain appropriate tests.

A competent physician will then outline these tests—X-rays and other special examinations that he recommends to help him arrive at a more specific diagnosis. He is looking for the underlying cause—the disease responsible for your diarrhea. He will explain the nature, risks, and costs of these examinations and, if you've agreed to have them, he will make an appointment for you and ask you to return later for a second evaluation.

While waiting for the results of these tests, it is proper for your doctor to start you on a drug in an effort to control your uncomfortable symptoms until he can make his diagnosis. This is not the same as if he were treating only your symptoms.

There is nothing mysterious about the diagnostic process carried out by the conscientious physician and you should feel a part of it. It takes time and effort. It involves an interview, an examination, a discussion, a scheduling of special tests and a reevaluation.

One very good sign that you're in proper hands and have little to fear is a frank admission by your doctor that he is uncertain of the cause of your problem and will have to perform several exams and possibly call in another consultant. This should not be misunderstood as a sign of professional weakness. If you expect your doctor to know it all, or if he is putting on an act, someone's in for a shock. The body is an extremely complicated machine, and the more we learn about it, the more we realize how vast is our ignorance. There is no room for overconfidence here and the humble doctor is a far wiser and more prudent professional than the doctor who appears to know it all.

If these things aren't happening, it's time for you to ask questions. Suppose the doctor listens only briefly to your symptoms of diarrhea, barely examines you, and dashes off a prescription—the whole operation lasting but ten minutes. This should arouse your curiosity. He is either a genius or simply irresponsible, and the odds are strong it's the latter. At best, you're being shortchanged; at worst, seriously damaged. Ask him what is causing the diarrhea. If he says "a virus" or "your nerves" (favorite ploys), ask him how he knows that? How did he come to that conclusion? Ask him if he's certain you don't have some serious disease. If he hedges (and he will), ask him if there aren't certain tests that might be carried out to give him (and you) more certainty.

Once you start pushing, you'll see his defenses start crumbling. He isn't familiar with this type of questioning from a patient and handles it poorly. He'll become exasperated, even angry, and blow his professional cool. This works, believe me, and is a sure sign that you've made a bad choice.

I am not encouraging a confrontation with every doctor. Nor am I suggesting that you start your relationship this way. **A**

conscientious physician will pursue a vigorous evaluation of your symptoms. Give him a chance, but judge him carefully.

2. Missing silent disease

Some diseases remain silent for a long time. The sooner they are detected, the better off you are. You don't get early warning symptoms.

But how can these latent diseases be detected if they cause no symptoms? The plain fact is that since we're not magicians or crystal-ball gazers, we can't always detect silent disease as early as we would wish. But we have to try and we're often successful. That's why we recommend physical examinations even for the healthy patient without symptoms. And that's why an examination is not complete if it's limited to only your complaints or symptoms: **Every encounter with your physician must include a thorough search for silent disease**. If he is diligent and thorough, he will often uncover far more serious problems than your symptoms suggest—and often the disease he uncovers may have nothing to do with your symptoms.

Suppose a woman visits her physician because of a headache. He makes a cursory examination and detects a mild form of high blood pressure. This might be an adequate explanation for the headache, and the woman returns in a month, happy to be relieved of her headaches. She leaves his office with her pills, pays his fee, and is told to return if the headaches recur.

But she also leaves with a large, undetected lump in her left breast. She will not know it's there for six more months. And the longer it goes undetected, the poorer her chance of surviving if it turns out to be cancerous. She then discovers the lump while bathing, delays a month out of anxiety, and finally seeks her physician's advice. When he discovers the lump, now quite large, he is liable to bawl her out for waiting a month. "Don't you realize how dangerous it is to wait so long with a breast lump?"

Wait a minute! Why wasn't this lump detected six months ago when she was in his office with a headache? Because he was too busy to examine her breasts? Because that's not what she was complaining about?

Nonsense, a good doctor would have given this woman a complete physical examination on her first visit. He would have found the lump, a far more threatening problem than her headaches. Had there been no detectable lump at that time, a good doctor, also being a good teacher, would have taught the woman the importance and technique of self-examination of the breasts. After that it would be her task to carry out these examinations at monthly intervals. A screening mammogram is also done at regular intervals even in the absence of a detectable lump.

We can't find all silent diseases—we will miss some—and I must emphasize this. But you can depend upon the principle: **Doctors miss silent diseases in proportion to how limited their examinations are.**

It is not reasonable to expect your doctor to repeat a one-hour examination on each visit. Such complete examinations should be carried out annually or when you are a new patient.

So you be the judge. Ask yourself:

Has my physician carried out a thorough examination?
Has he looked for silent diseases?
Does he limit his examination to only those areas which I complain about?

If you accept the premise that certain diseases cause no symptoms for a long period of time **(the latent period)**, then common sense tells you that a doctor who only listens to your symptoms and restricts his examination to this area of your anatomy is going to miss far more silent disease than a physician who is willing to turn over every stone in his search for disease. You should find it reassuring, and a good indicator of your doctor's competency, when he searches for diseases on the slightest provocation.

Let me give you one more example. Let's suppose you are seeking medical attention for chest pain of four week's duration and you have chosen a new doctor and are anxious about his competency. In addition to asking questions obviously relevant to your chest symptoms, this physician reviews all your organ systems, past history, family history and social history. He examines your chest and does a complete physical examination as I described earlier.

This sequence should be very reassuring. It is an excellent indication of competence and, providing all other indicators described in this book are present, you are in the hands of a good doctor. He is working hard at evaluating your health, and is unlikely to miss silent disease.

3. Failure to recognize early signs of serious disease.

Silent disease may be impossible to detect for a long period of time. But there comes a point when subtle changes occur, when the underlying pathology breaks through and early signs of the disease become manifest. A good doctor is always on the alert for these subtle changes. He pursues every symptom in detail, never writing them off as, "It's a virus that's prevalent," or "It's probably just your nerves." **He thoroughly explores any abnormality he finds during your physical examination until he finds an adequate explanation.** If you wonder, at times, why he's putting you through such extensive tests at the slightest sign of trouble, it's because he is a good doctor and does not wish to overlook early signs of serious disease. **A wise old G.P. put it this way, "A diagnosis at any price."**

Contrast this with the physician who continuously brushes off your symptoms, telling you it's all in your head. He is usually just as casual with his examination, rarely doing a complete one. You will be able to detect his blasé attitude after one or two visits.

This failure to recognize the early signs of serious disease may be disastrous for you. Fortunately, there is often a second chance and you should not let things happen this way again. This is where the principle comes in that a good doctor works hard at diagnosis. If you find yourself in the throes of a serious disease, whatever it may be, ask yourself whether your physician ought to have discovered it earlier. How many times have you seen him in the past year or two? For what reasons? Did he do a thorough examination and question you about your general health in any of these visits? Or, rather, did he give you the five-minute visit and the pat on the shoulder. Did he ever attempt to educate you about your health, the general measures you should take to improve it, things you should correct that lead to bad health? **A good doctor constantly tries to teach the art of healthy living to his patients.**

You must never blame "bad luck" for your illness, until you have thoroughly questioned the responsibility of your physician. Again, in fairness to the medical profession, we are not fortune-tellers and cannot guarantee or even predict good health. Many illnesses strike with no warning, and the best diagnostician in the world cannot certify good health. But the doctor is your health counselor and must take prime responsibility for early detection of serious disease. Failure to recognize the early signs of serious disease, when coupled with a pattern of practice which includes rapid interviews and incomplete examinations, is a sign of a poor physician.

4. Making telephone diagnoses.

All the bad habits of sloppy medical practice converge in the still-too-common practice of diagnosing illness by phone and prescribing drugs without seeing the patient. There are rare occasions when a patient may benefit from a telephone diagnosis. For example, when a patient's illness is well known to his doctor, a telephone diagnosis may save an unnecessary office visit. **But in the vast majority of cases, diagnoses over the telephone border on malpractice**. If your doctor makes a habit of such a practice, you should dismiss him immediately.

If you have paid attention to what I have been saying, the reason for my harsh criticism of telephone diagnoses should be immediately evident. It can't be done! Fancy telephonic audio-visual communications which link electrocardiographic tracings and paramedical personnel to experts in medical emergency centers are a different situation entirely, and I am not referring to this. What I call telephone diagnosing is that practice, typical of a busy, harried or sloppy doctor who, rather than spend time examining his patients, merely guesses at the cause of their trouble without seeing them and, on the strength of this guess and reliance on the laws of chance, prescribes a medicine and tells them to call back in a day or two if they feel worse. This is not responsible medical practice and indicates a callous attitude.

5. Using dangerous drugs unnecessarily.

Serious, even fatal, drug reactions are a very common experience in modern medical practice. The drugs available to physicians today are extremely potent because they have the ability to alter your physiological state. That's what makes them good drugs. This was not so sixty to eighty years ago. Most of the old tonic waters and herb medicines were innocuous but not very effective. Very few people developed complications from sarsaparilla root but it probably didn't do any good either. With the advent of pharmacologically active drugs, the entire picture has changed. **Drugs now actually cause more disability and death than major surgery.**

A responsible physician uses powerful drugs with great caution, and only when absolutely necessary. The majority of acute illnesses are self-limited and, given enough time, resolve themselves. In the case of some drugs, the cure can be worse than the disease. Before prescribing drugs, the physician must try his best to arrive at a precise diagnosis and give only that amount of the drug necessary to effect a cure.

Antibiotics are among the most abused drugs in modern medicine. They are effective only against bacterial infections. Many respiratory infections, including common colds and sore throats, are due to viruses for which antibiotics are of no value. They have to run their course for four or five days; little can be done to speed the healing process. The physician, anxious to look like he's doing something, may prescribe an antibiotic for a viral infection. Unfortunately, severe and even fatal penicillin reactions do occur each year, making such treatment totally unacceptable. Before prescribing an antibiotic, the physician must first prove that the infection is susceptible to the antibiotic and this usually requires sending sputum, blood or other fluid specimens for bacteriological study. This is called *taking a culture.*

I have mentioned antibiotics because they are so commonly used and because their misuse is also too common. But I could make the same point with cardiac drugs, water pills, weight-reducing medicines, tranquilizers and other drugs. When used properly, they are effective agents. Used unnecessarily or improperly, they can be very dangerous. **If your doctor is competent, he will not place you on a medication without telling you its name, what he is using it for, what risks attend its use and what early warning signs you should look for.**

A physician who has taken the time to explain everything you need to know about the drug he is prescribing is not likely to prescribe unnecessarily. He obviously has a healthy respect for the potency of the drug, which is why he spends the time to go over its risks with you.

Contrast this with the doctor who hands you a barely legible prescription and tells you simply to follow the directions and to "come back in a month." You walk out of his office unaware of the name of the drug, its purpose, its risks, or its side effects.

I am amazed how many patients are so willing to take drugs without knowing what the risks are. It's their blind faith that is responsible for a large number of tragedies. If your doctor keeps you in the dark about the drugs he prescribes, he may also prescribe the drugs unnecessarily.

Never take a drug, the name, nature, risks and side effects of which are not clearly spelled out to you by your physician.

6. Under-therapy.

Insecure physicians often prescribe less than the accepted dose of a drug. Under-therapy can lead to grave problems simply because the disease is not adequately treated. Since a great part of the doctor's usefulness to his patients is in the area of drug therapy, it makes no sense for him to be so insecure that he constantly undertreats his patients.

I have no easy rule for you to detect under-therapy. We are dealing with clinical judgment. And the physician, in this case a rather insecure one, has judged that the dangers of the drug outweigh the dangers of the disease; hence his hesitancy to prescribe properly. The dangers are somewhat reduced, however, if the physician is otherwise thorough and conscientious about his examinations and follows his patients carefully. If, on the other hand, he is an insecure physician who undertreats and under-examines his patient, then the combination can be lethal and you had best have it out with him. **Always discuss the drug and its dosage with your physician. The very fact that you ask about this often influences his management for the better.**

7. Over-therapy.

Over-therapy is an uncommon practice among incompetent physicians. Even a callous doctor is sensible enough to realize that, given the decision to use a drug, it is safer to under-use than to over-use it. He probably has enough horse sense to stay away from powerful drugs or at least use them in less than adequate dosages. Rarely will he prescribe an overdose of such drugs. But it can happen, of course.

A variant of the overdose problem is the incompetent doctor's failure to recognize that you are already taking a drug that exaggerates the effect of the drug he is now prescribing. The best advice I can give you about avoiding an over-dosage is simply to be sure that your doctor carries on an intelligent and thorough discussion with you about the drug he is prescribing. This is always your best protection against the dangers of drugs. Some physicians have a fetish about keeping their patients in the dark about the drugs they are taking. They seem to feel that the mystery is part of the treatment.

8. Not recognizing early drug reactions.

Every drug is capable of causing serious, even fatal, reactions. The warning signs may be obvious or very subtle. The physician who fails to warn you about these possible side effects has no respect for the dangers of modern drugs and is unlikely to recognize early warning signs himself. In fact, you are the only effective monitor of early warning signs of a drug reaction, but to monitor them intelligently you have to be told what to watch for.

Some drugs cause one or two side reactions; others can cause dozens of symptoms. A conscientious doctor will either discuss this with you or, better still, give you a printout listing all of the possible symptoms that you should anticipate. **An intelligent thing for you to do is to ask your doctor for a written list of these possible drug reactions**. If he refuses to comply and doesn't at least discuss the reactions with you, you're in dangerous hands and ought to seek another doctor's advice. If the computer is friendly for you, ask it to tell you about drug reactions.

Suppose you are taking a drug and develop a new set of symptoms, symptoms that weren't part of your original illness. **You should contact your physician immediately!** He may be quite familiar with these symptoms and recognize them as not serious. But he may have to examine you before he can make that determination. If he takes your anxiety too casually, be on the alert and insist on some reassurance that it is not a serious drug reaction.

9. Recommending surgery too early.

Unnecessary surgery occurs. Incompetent doctors often jump the gun, so to speak, and recommend operations prematurely. I discuss this and other aspects of unnecessary surgery in chapter 15.

10. Recommending surgery too late.

Some doctors have so much professional pride that they withhold surgery in a futile effort to cure the disease with drugs. Often this is just as bad as recommending surgery too early. But this is becoming less and less of a problem as physicians specialize more and more and are quick to recognize the need for a second opinion about surgical intervention. The modern physician, regardless of whatever other failings he may have, is quick to recognize when a surgeon should be called. As a surgeon, I find less and less tendency on the part of physicians to call me too late.

11. Failure to consult with another specialist

Pride, more than ignorance, is at the root of this potentially fatal error of the incompetent doctor. He simply never realizes his own shortcomings. The human body is far too complex to be understood by any one physician. **Even Einstein did not understand the whole universe.**

If you ever feel your physician is stuck for a diagnosis or what to do next for therapy, ask him whether a second opinion or a consultation with another specialist is in order. If you get the resistance vibe, analyze it very carefully. It often indicates arrogance and pride of the inadequate doctor who fears a different opinion from a colleague.

If this happens more than a few times in your relationship with your doctor, it is time to make for the road and seek a different primary care doctor.

12. Not managing several specialists.

At times, especially during a complicated hospitalization, your physician must call in several specialists to examine you. For example, you're recovering from a major operation or injury and are in cardiac and kidney failure. At the same time your lungs fill up with fluid. Here your doctor may have to call in a cardiologist, a nephrologist and a pulmonologist.

To make matters worse, a major infection takes hold of your already depleted immune system during this serious illness and on comes an infectious disease expert to add to the mix of doctors managing your case.

The problem is this. With so many cooks handling the soup, problems arise. There can be duplications of drugs; inadvertent use of incompatible drugs; parts of the illness that overlap; where two or three specialists feel the problem belongs to the other doctor, coverage problems which worsen at night or on weekends.

Doctors don't readily admit to these mix-ups and so the public (that is YOU) rarely hear about them or seem to think all this is far-fetched. Trust me, it happens more than you think and more than we doctors like to admit.

The best analogy I can offer is the exact reason a large symphony orchestra, no matter how skilled the individual musician, needs an orchestra conductor to pull the whole thing together. **Your primary care physician is your orchestra conductor. This job can never be relegated to a flutist or a violinist, a cardiologist or a kidney specialist.**

13. Rationing the physician's availability.

This chapter talks about bad things incompetent doctors do that threaten your health. Some of the problems are not the doctor's direct fault. Rationing of care, provoked by health insurance systems and HMOs, is a dangerous new trend in medicine, one of the thirteen things that can kill you.

I am referring to the roadblocks that insurance systems and HMOs place in your way to reduce the availability of your physician to you. Try calling your doctor at night. After you get through the "dial 1 if you have a bill to be paid; dial 2 if you have an insurance problem," etc, then watch how they throw paramedics and physician assistants in your way to avoid the more expensive physician talking to you.

Time Out!

"OK," you say, "I am a patient, not a physician or a disease expert. How in the world am I to tell if I am being over- or undertreated, if surgery has been recommended too soon or too late, if a serious disease should have been detected earlier? Please, this all sounds like fantasy to me."

Hold on. Reread the above chapter carefully. Reread all the previous chapters in this book. No, you are not a physician and not expected to know all these dangerous signs of the incompetent physician. You are required, and it is surely within your intellectual reach, to ask intelligent questions, ask them frequently, **give thought to what is going on.**

Example: If your physician sends you to a surgeon and he says surgery is not necessary— "bingo." This one experience does not make a case against your primary-care physician, but it requires that you ask the surgeon why he differs from your physician and then go over things again with your physician. Try to ascertain whether his view is just a sincere difference of opinion or whether he should have known better in the first place.

If you were not examined for a lump in your breast and, four months later, you're told the lump should have been found earlier—"bingo."

Each of these failures can be recognized in time, but only if you make a serious effort to understand, to question your doctor, to get second opinions, to give each and every experience with your doctor some very serious thought.

Don't just assume he or she is infallible and let it go without question.

Chapter 13: The Doctor as a Responsible Professional

"is there a REAL doctor in the house"?

Chapter summary: This chapter begins to show you some of the tragic problems developing in our health care system because the insurance companies and their number crunchers have taken control of the doctor's schedule. This is **flee-from-service**. The doctor becomes inaccessible, tired, rushed, disconnected from you, her patient. I attempt to summarize what professionalism is all about and some of the truly great problems affecting modern medicine and detracting from a true professionalism that is vital in the doctor-patient relationship. We shall begin to see how you can manage this situation.

I've tried to give some basic principles by which you can judge your doctor's competency. I have mentioned the value of a good reputation, the importance of a doctor's caring, why teaching is the essence of good medical care, and various ways in which you can judge how hard she works at solving your problems. I also described thirteen common practice faults of poor physicians.

But there is more to good doctoring than a general statement about caring and a list of do's and don'ts. A good physician is a responsible professional. Responsibility implies a totality of caring, a never-ending process. It is not a 9-to-5 job. Medicine just cannot work that way. **The first sign of a responsible doctor is his availability and accessibility**.

How long should it take to get an appointment for a routine visit with a physician? That depends on what you mean by a "routine" visit. If you're feeling perfectly well and simply wish to be scheduled for an annual check-up, quite possibly you will have to wait several weeks. This may be inconvenient, but you will learn to schedule this type of examination well in advance.

But what about the forty-two year old woman who found a lump in her left breast two weeks ago? She has been absolutely petrified about her discovery; so much so that she has been frozen in inaction for two weeks, unable to get up the courage to call her doctor, each night hoping that it will go away, only to wake up in the morning to find the lump still present. She is afraid to tell her husband about it and embarrassed to discuss it with her friends. **You cannot comprehend how isolated she feels, unless you have had the same experience.**

The reaction is universal. First there is a period of total disbelief. This may go on for two or three weeks. She just can't believe this could happen and almost convinces herself that it's just a swelling from an injury and will surely go away. Then follows a period of inaction—a total inability to do anything about it. She cannot talk or think about it. This may last a few unbearable days and is natural and human.

Given this state of mind, how should the doctor respond when this woman finally gets up the courage to call her? Any doctor who is genuinely concerned for her patients, who cares about them as people—who is a responsible professional—should consider this an emergency situation and **make room for the patient the day she calls**. She may not be expected to do a complete physical the same day, but she ought to examine her breast, decide what has to be done, and go on from there. Quite frequently what the patient thinks is a breast lump turns out to be no lump at all and the tremendous psychological strain can be relieved in a minute or two by the simple act of reassurance.

What are we to say about a physician who is brusque in this hour of human need and tells the patient that her first appointment opening is in two weeks? Or, still worse, the physician who gives her secretary the job of telling the patient: **"The doctor can squeeze you in, two weeks from next Thursday."**

It is highly unlikely that a two-week delay will alter this woman's chances of a cure should the lump turn out to be cancer. Looked at scientifically, the doctor cannot be faulted for asking this patient to wait two weeks. But consider what a two-week wait does to the patient. It has already taken this woman two weeks to get up the courage to make an appointment. Now she is being asked to live alone with her anguish an additional two weeks. Such a situation, from a humane point of view, is positively inexcusable. **The woman should be seen on the day she places the phone call!** And in my judgment a doctor who hasn't got the instinct to understand this and to instruct her secretary accordingly is either callous beyond recall, overextended to the point of becoming a less-than-adequate physician, or just does not care about her patients and will not come through consistently in a tight situation. **She may be an excellent scientific medical technician but she is not a good doctor.**

I have no use for the defenders of the profession who would minimize the importance of such an irresponsible act by claiming that the doctor wasn't malicious, that she just didn't realize the emotional impact. A responsible physician would recognize that impact.

How do you define "Availability"?

The responsible physician is accessible for physical as well as psychological emergencies and must, throughout her active practice life, accept the viewpoint that her convenience must be sacrificed again and again when her patient's well-being hangs in the balance.

Availability is very relative but difficult to define. You will have to make your own judgment. Does your doctor put you off with postponed appointments? If so, how often? Is she always on some "emergency," thereby inconveniencing you and upsetting your plans? How long do you wait in her office to see her? Can you get her on nights and weekends? Is she always signed out to someone else who, in turn, is not readily available? What about her vacation coverage? Are you satisfied that the physician left to cover her practice is equally competent and available?

Can you talk with your doctor by telephone or does her secretary consistently protect her from you? Does she return your calls when she can't be reached by telephone? Or do you have to keep trying and wonder whether her answering service or secretary ever gave her your message?

Don't underestimate the importance of availability. Some physicians are excellent when you are dealing with them face-to-face but damned hard to reach between visits. They seem to limit their responsibility to their immediate patients as if responsibility were a part- time preoccupation. Emergencies strike unpredictably and you should feel secure that your personal physician is easily accessible when you need her. Being unable to reach your garage mechanic in off hours is an aggravation. But if you cannot discuss your medical emergencies during off hours, weekends or holidays, then harm can come to you since your doctor knows your problem best and can handle an emergency better than some strange doctor in an emergency room.

Who's minding the store?

Your doctor will need to take time off, of course, for relaxation, her family, postgraduate education, and so on. Years ago the old-time family doctor was available seven days a week, nights and holidays. At least that's the image people have of her. It may have been so, but it was not a wholesome situation—a family doctor on call seven days a week, nights and holidays was a fatigued, strained physician who could not function properly. Time off is essential; therefore you will occasionally have to settle for your doctor's substitute.

A good doctor invariably signs off to an equally competent physician. Her substitute does not know every detail of your case and will obviously have a different personality, different pace, and a different approach. But this isn't necessarily bad. It gives you a chance to compare your regular physician to this new one. You may even find that you like this doctor's style better than your own physician's!

You should not have to be inconvenienced just because your doctor has taken time off. You should feel as secure in the hands of her associate as you do with her. Although there is no way to schedule major illness, you should not have to suffer just because illness strikes while your doctor is on vacation. **Your physician is responsible for leaving you with competent coverage**. If the covering physician is not readily available, you ought to discuss the matter with your doctor on her return. She may not be fully aware of the coverage habits of her partner or associate.

Do I know you?

A responsible physician knows her patients thoroughly as individuals. Some of this knowledge is stored in her memory and can be recalled without any effort. Much of it is stored in the medical record which is always available when she is examining or interviewing you. **But whichever method she chooses, you can sense that she knows your case.** When you visit her a second or third time, ask yourself how aware she seems to be about your case. Does she clearly recall the problems you discussed on your last visit? Does she keep records and refer to them with each visit? You can be reassured if she has these records available during your visit and refers to them. It means she cares enough about your problem not to trust memory but to commit certain facts to a written record so that she can refresh her memory from time to time.

With a good doctor you sense a continuity of care from one visit to another. She brings together any loose ends. You don't have to keep reminding her of "the three problems" she's supposed to check. If your doctor frequently seems to cover up her oversights you can sense it if you know what to look for. Don't underestimate the value of these lapses as indicators of competence.

Let us suppose that you saw Dr. Jones two months ago and your major complaints were (1) heartburn and (2) a small lump in your groin. During her examination, she also found a small, dark mole along your belt line which she felt should be removed once she had thoroughly evaluated your heartburn problem.

The lump in the groin turned out to be a hernia for which she recommended surgery but, again, only after she had evaluated the heartburn. So you have three problems: (1) undiagnosed heartburn, (2) a small hernia, and (3) a pigmented mole. She sends you for a series of X-rays and a gastric ulcer is discovered. She telephones you as soon as the X-ray report is available **(a sign of a responsible doctor**). She tells you about the ulcer and recommends whatever she feels is appropriate to heal it. She also tells you to come back in one month so she can see if the treatment is effective. At that time she will also put you through a thorough educational program about the nature of ulcer disease.

You're back in a month and feeling fine. The heartburn has been completely relieved and you're ready to return to a completely normal life.

A good doctor keeps good records. Without having to be reminded, she now discusses your hernia and the pigmented mole, tying loose ends together. She again recommends that the hernia be repaired and, if she deems it necessary, that the mole be removed. With your approval, she refers you to a surgeon and asks that you return after the surgery has been done. She takes it upon herself to inform the surgeon that you have an ulcer, that it is well controlled and that it ought not to cause any problem in the post operative period. While you are in the hospital, she drops in for a social visit (for which she usually does not charge a fee) and, if necessary, advises the surgeon about any other problems he may anticipate.

How different this is from an irresponsible physician. She sends you for the same set of X-rays and you never hear from her. So you call, quite anxious about the results. Her secretary informs you that "doctor is busy" and then tells you that the X-ray showed an ulcer and that you should come back for another visit. On your second visit, you are handed a diet and given some medication to take. No further mention is made of the hernia or the mole. So you remind the doctor about these two problems. There is a short pause. She hadn't remembered those two problems. "Oh yes," she says, "well, you ought to have them taken care of. I don't do surgery. Why don't you choose a surgeon and go see him?" Somehow you pick a surgeon, make an appointment and are advised to have the hernia repaired and the mole removed. You are hospitalized and the surgeon asks about your general health. You are surprised that he doesn't know about your ulcer. "Didn't Dr. Jones talk with you?" you ask. "No, she didn't," the surgeon replies. The surgery is done. Dr. Jones is glad to hear you recovered. But no, she couldn't drop by to see you. She was busy and you didn't need her. There were no problems—just a routine hernia repair.

Which of these two doctors is a responsible professional? Both have excellent credentials. Both can pass any certifying examination. Who is to judge? A consumer-advocacy group? A government-certifying agent?

I submit that only you can judge which is a good doctor, that only you are in a position to evaluate such indicators as

responsibility, care, teaching, thoroughness, reliability and follow-through.

Here are two doctors who detect the same problems—an ulcer, hernia and pigmented mole. They both recommend an X-ray to confirm the ulcer, an anti-ulcer regimen, and surgery for the hernia and mole. Their standards for treatment are identical, but their approaches to patient care are totally different. **That's what makes the difference between a doctor who is professional and one who isn't.**

A few more clues:

Being a responsible professional implies even more. I have written at some length about a physician's thoroughness as an indicator of quality and will emphasize it again. Is your doctor thorough in her examinations? Does she do a pap smear, looking for cervical cancer whenever she does a pelvic examination? The only way to know is to ask her. Does she routinely do rectal examinations during your annual physical examinations? **Thoroughness counts!**

What about professional pride? It can be an asset when it leads to thoroughness but a liability when it leads to smugness and a know-it-all attitude. **There is no such thing as an all-around expert in modern medicine. With today's knowledge explosion, the wizard doctor no longer exists.**

How well does your doctor keep up with developments in modern medicine? How often does she take postgraduate courses? Does she ever mention them to you? When it seems appropriate, ask how she manages to keep up with developments in medicine. Has she ever said that she would like to consult with another physician about managing your case? Has she ever referred you to a medical center for another opinion? Does she seem overconfident, always sure that she has the answer? Have you ever asked her about getting another opinion on a difficult problem, only to receive an arrogant reply, "I don't need another opinion on your case," or something like that? No one knows the answers to all medical problems, so **it is a good sign when a physician says that she would like to get another opinion.**

A good doctor is humble enough to admit her limitations. Her mind is open, not closed and immovable. She is responsible to you and manifests it in a number of ways. She willingly and enthusiastically takes responsibility for your care. She doesn't pass the buck. When things go wrong, as they sometimes do, she acknowledges her share of responsibility; she doesn't blame you or some other physician.

Beware of false decorum, the excessively professionalized doctor. She wears the white coat, carries a stethoscope hung neatly around her neck, and uses technical terms to confuse you. You can tell how seriously she takes her job by observing her decorum and that of her staff. How well does she follow through with your problems? How seriously does she view your concerns? Does she seem truly interested or is she putting on an air of gravity. **The mark of a self-confident and emotionally well-balanced physician is that she appears to be a real person**

If she is good, she will have a wholesome relationship with her patients. She will be warm and close, not austere and distant. She will be neither condescending nor demeaning but will carry on an adult-to-adult relationship.

The ultimate sign of a responsible professional is how dependable she is when the chips are down. Does she come through at the right time? Where was she when you needed her most? **Can you trust her when your life depends on it?**

Time Out!

Once again, all this seems a fantasy in this modern world of rush, rationing, restriction. Doctors are handcuffed by giant HMOs and health insurance schemes to render as little expensive care as they can, to use specialists very sparingly if at all, to hold back on hospitalization, and on and on it goes.

This is all very true and very regrettable. In the long run I believe the public will reject this rationing of their care and this blockage between doctor and patient. In the short run you must do the fighting for your own well-being.

The fight starts when you first realize that you are being held back from even talking to your doctor. She is made unavailable, invisible to you precisely because her services are too expensive for the insurance companies. They prefer to have you consult with a paramedic or a nurse practitioner, wonderful professionals but not your doctor. **All you have to do to force the magical appearance of your doctor on the telephone or in**

person is to demand to see him or her. Demand it or threaten to report the HMO to the state Medical Society. Always add that you will contact the better business bureau or some consumer agency; also add that you plan to contact your local newspaper. Always follow through with these threats. They will help you and all patients who happen to be enlisted in your HMO.

Trust me, these methods get immediate results.

Chapter 14: Let's Talk Money

"pulse vs. purse"

Chapter Summary: What are reasonable fees for medical services? How are you to judge them? What can you do if you feel you have been fleeced by your physician? Read on.

Once I frantically drove my car into a small auto repair shop in a secluded midwestern town. I had heard a terrible cranking noise in the engine and could smell something burning. Knowing nothing about engines, I thought the whole thing was falling apart. A two-minute check by the mechanic uncovered a bare wire which was short circuiting something in the generator. He repaired the problem in two minutes and everything was like new. I feared the worst when I asked him how much, knowing I was at the mercy of both my own ignorance about engines and a strange mechanic in a small town. He told me to forget it. There was no charge. I insisted that he take something for his time, work and judgment, but he refused and laughed it off.

There is a certain decency about a professional man's work and a certain reasonable relationship between what he does and what he charges. How much was this auto mechanic justified in charging? He could have charged me a portion of an hour's work, some odd part of, say, fifty dollars. Or he could have looked at it as a vital job done in a pinch, saving me the inconvenience of finding another mode of transportation. Then he could have charged me an arm and a leg. But he was decent and decided, given the trivial nature of the repair, that it was better to consider it a favor. He had a sense of balance about the business side of his profession. He sensed that it would all come out in the wash.

Was this man a hayseed, a decent person, a fool, or just not caught up in the crass commercialism of urban life? A little bit of all of these probably and that's what you have to look for in your doctor. I can't tell you what's a reasonable fee for a given service (there are so many intangibles), but I can tell you that your physician should be decent in his billing. Has he ever done anything for you without charge, or does he "nickel and dime" you for everything? This is not a trivial question. It tells what your doctor's real values are. Does he serve you because that is his responsibility as a physician or because he can collect a fee for every service performed?

You're convalescing from a major operation. Your primary physician drops by the hospital to see you once or twice. He doesn't render any specific professional service; at least you have no grounds to believe that he is actively involved in your care. Does he bill you for "two hospital visits" —May 12 and May 13? Technically, he could easily justify his visits on the ground that he was supporting your surgeon, advising him about your cardiac status, for example. If that is what he actually did, the bill is quite appropriate. **But has it ever happened that he didn't charge for something he did?** A social visit at the hospital? Like the auto mechanic, there is really no decent way he could charge. That's what you should look for, little signs that indicate that your doctor isn't all hung up on fees-for-services—on making a buck.

The cost of medical care is soaring rapidly, perhaps more than most other costs in our society. Much of the increase is in hospital, drug and nursing home costs, although physicians' fees amount to about 20 percent of national health expenditures.

You should understand before you're treated just how expensive your doctor is and how he wishes to be paid. Not all fees are paid by third-party insurers like Blue Shield. Co-payments seem to be on the rise. You should inquire about routine fees for office and hospital visits. You should know the fee for any special procedure your doctor wishes to perform. You may feel embarrassed to bring up the subject. The result is a standoff. If neither you nor your doctor talk about fees there may be misunderstandings which will lead to trouble later.

Your best solution may be to talk to the doctor's secretary or nurse. She will be able to tell you what he charges. Indeed, she will probably know more about his fees and what part medical insurance pays than the doctor does. **Be certain to talk to either the doctor or his staff about money and find out in advance how much his services are going to cost**.

Suppose a doctor is too expensive for your pocketbook yet you would like to remain his patient. I can almost guarantee that if you approach him and speak frankly about your economic limitations, he will make special arrangements to continue seeing you. In fact, this would be an excellent indicator of his sense of decency. Conversely, if he tells you to get lost or puts you off some other way, he's the kind of mercenary I've been talking about. Better not darken his doorway again.

Modern medicine appears to have gone where the money is—a tragic turn. It is difficult to figure out what went wrong. In my most critical moments, I believe that we physicians have just become too mercenary, trying to extract every last cent for the services we render. Then I think of the alternative—government-salaried physicians, unproductive civil servants who worry more about tenure and security than taking care of their patients. In my more charitable moments, I believe that we physicians are victims of the same commercial mentality that affects other sectors of society. No profession is immune to the scramble for dollars.

A particularly disastrous trend—one which physicians helped create—is the rise of third-party payment mechanisms: Blue Shield, Blue Cross, Medicare, Medicaid, HMO insurance systems. Practically everything we physicians do is partly paid for by one of these insurers. This alters the relationship between a doctor and his patient. It forces him to spend almost as much time filling out forms as caring for patients. **What is more, certain technical procedures pay much more than counseling, so doctors tend to spend a great deal of time on technical services rather than counseling or teaching patients**. Most health insurance companies pay an excellent fee for a five-minute minor operation but may pay nothing for an hour's discussion with a patient or his family. This shouldn't influence how we physicians spend our time, I know, but although few doctors will admit it, the natural inclination is to go where the money is.

Since we're stuck with the ethics of our times, we might as well make the best of it until some social genius unglues the whole mess. Let's see if we can distinguish less greedy doctors from the rest of the pack and find out how they differ.

A doctor is both a professional man and a businessman. He must strike a happy balance between his professional responsibilities and his business obligations. Unfortunately, there is little room in modern society for the idealist, the "Hippocrates" who would minister to the sick regardless of their ability to pay. Practicing medicine is an enormously expensive undertaking and bills have to be paid. Government regulations, malpractice insurance, employees' salaries and mundane things such as rent, utility bills and automobile expenses, are the realities of business life that affect the practice of medicine like everything else.

Contrary to what you might think, the average doctor does not "make a killing," although he does have a higher income than many other entrepreneurs in our society. It is precisely because of this high income and the critical nature of his work that he incurs a greater obligation to go easier with his bill than other businessmen.

Suppose you receive a bill that is excessively large, one not in keeping with his usual practice. What should you do? Drop in and discuss it with him or his secretary. Inquiries about bills are common; there won't be any hard feelings. It may be a simple error by a secretary or an oversight on the doctor's part. This has happened to me a number of times and I have often found, much to my embarrassment, that it was either my mistake or my staff's.

I cannot tell you when a bill is unreasonable. You will have to judge that by your own experience. But suppose, for the sake of the argument, that you have been ripped off. What can you do about it?

The worst thing you can do is pay the bill and grin and bear it! This does your pocketbook no good and doesn't help your neighbor who might feel the sting next.

First, call the doctor's office and politely but firmly request an explanation. It could be a simple mistake. But suppose it isn't— that's just what the doctor charges for his services. Tell him or his secretary that you're not about to pay the bill, that you think it is unreasonable and want an explanation.

If they explain the bill, you will have to judge its validity. But suppose they refuse to discuss it with you or you simply won't accept the explanation. What next?

There are several ways to handle this situation. The easiest way, but not the best, is simply to tear up each subsequent monthly bill. Most physicians won't chase you. If a bill collector calls or comes to your home, explain why you haven't paid the bill and refuse him too. That should end the matter. If the doctor does pursue that matter and you end up in small-claims court (**a most unlikely event**), the judge will attempt to find a responsible compromise and nothing more.

The best way to handle an inordinate bill is to write a polite but firm letter to your state medical society. Describe the physician's services and include a copy of his bill. If he is a surgeon, his bill will usually include the name of the operation. Estimate how long he worked on you, tell what he did, what he said he did, and so on. Describe how you have attempted to discuss the matter and how he responded. Include a clear and polite warning that you expect prompt action by the medical society and, failing this, you will report the matter to the state consumer-protection agency or your attorney. Send a copy of your letter to the doctor who billed you so that he will know what action you have taken and what your plans are. **Always consider a copy to your local newspaper!**

Analyze your tactics carefully before you act. First, review the circumstances under which I have advocated sending a letter to the medical society. Don't be rash or unfair. Make a reasonable effort to discuss the situation with your doctor. And be as sure as you can that the fee really is outlandish. If you can't do this, go by your instincts or experiences—judge the bill according to how long the doctor worked on you and how much effort he went to compared with your experience with other doctors.

In your letter to the medical society be sure to state that you do not intend to let this matter rest. **Your letter will receive immediate attention— of that I can assure you.** Often, the medical society is looking for just this type of letter to bring pressure on a notorious bad apple against whom it has been powerless to act because it lacked a specific charge. Bad apples damage the reputation of the entire medical profession yet they are very difficult to control and even harder to eliminate.

After receiving your letter, the society's ethics or fees committee with sit down with the doctor and discuss the matter. If his bill is unreasonably high, they may pressure him to compromise. They may or may not succeed. They have no legal authority to force a doctor to lower his bill, but you can be sure that he will long remember this visit.

If you get no satisfaction from the medical society, send them a reminder of what you plan to do and, without further delay, write to a consumer-protection agency or take the matter to your attorney. **Under no circumstances should you feel obligated to pay any part of this bill.** A brief but well-thought-out letter to the editor of your local newspaper is perfectly appropriate and something I recommend. State the problem in specific and accurate detail. Say that you have received no response from the medical society. Be sure the society receives a copy of this letter!

I make these recommendations not to attack my profession but rather out of a firm conviction that it is my colleagues and I who are suffering from the occasional physician who gouges the public. There is no way members of the medical profession can single out these doctors and set their fees for them. Yet they damage all of us. If enough patients would do as I have recommended, the problem would be solved. So if you have a reasonable case, go to it and

happy hunting!

Time Out!

"Call a lawyer? Check with my local consumer protection agency? Sit down with my newspaper editor?"

"Go away! I am 79 years old and suffering from severe chronic illnesses which I cannot even name. I have no idea what my doctor does to me when I pay him a visit, let alone what a normal charge should be for these services!"

Hold on. Do you have a son or a daughter or a niece or a nephew? There has to be someone on your side when these financial crises arise. Don't hide behind your age or your illnesses. That's what families or relatives are for. Sit down with one of them and explain the problem in detail. You'll be surprised how much they owe you over a lifetime.

As I said, happy hunting.

Chapter 15: How to Avoid Surgery or at Least Live with It

"does your dog bite?"

Chapter summary: Some operations are more necessary than others, to paraphrase an old adage. This chapter attempts to deal with the media's frequent announcement that unnecessary surgery is going on all over the globe. Here I attempt to define unnecessary surgery, how it comes about and how you can often avoid it. Following a definition of "unnecessary," somewhat different from the print and television versions, I go on to give some very specific examples to show how the whole issue is very confusing and how best to avoid it in the first place. This is a critical chapter, especially in this age where, due to managed care planners, very necessary surgery is also often being curtailed or rationed.

Part of my message in this book is to warn readers about some of the shortcomings of the medical profession. Just as there are doctors who are responsible, competent, and personally concerned with their patients' welfare, there are doctors who are greedy, irresponsible, incompetent and impersonal. This is as true of surgical specialties as it is of medical and other specialties.

What is unnecessary surgery? Is it surgery for no reason other than profit? Perhaps the problem is widespread incompetence—bad calls and unnecessary operations. If so, what a grave indictment of the whole surgical educational process!

Surgeons spend many years in training, developing their judgment in fully certified residency programs. They are exposed to a wide variety of expert judgments by professional staffs in teaching hospitals. To qualify as surgeons, they must pass a rigorous selection process, designed to screen out those who lack judgment and skill. Would you expect this to produce many unnecessary surgical procedures? I do not believe that it has. I believe the residency concept and on-the-job training have produced excellent surgeons.

Then why the outcry about unnecessary surgery? I cannot reconcile my observations with reports in the media. The more I think about it, the more I suspect that the issue is philosophical.

Let me give an example. A 35 year-old woman wishes to have her varicose veins removed because she feels they are unsightly. She is not suffering any complications which make such surgery necessary. Her varicose veins aren't causing her any significant discomfort and they certainly are not disabling. She simply wants them removed because she does not like their appearance. Otherwise, she is in excellent health and should recover from surgery without difficulty. She understands the slight risk of the surgery and still wishes to proceed.

You might feel that varicose surgery is her business. Who are you to say whether or not she should undergo surgery simply for cosmetic purposes? But bear in mind that she probably has health insurance and some of the cost of her surgery will be passed on to you in the form of higher insurance premiums. Should you have anything to say about the surgery? Is the decision to operate exclusively the right of a consenting patient with a willing surgeon? Or should society, which pays the bill, have some say in the matter? And if society does have the right to enter into the decision, through what agency? **Should the insurance company, government, or some consumer-protection agency act on behalf of the public and prohibit certain forms of "unnecessary" surgery such as varicose veins, in order to reduce the overall cost of surgical care?**

People are truly concerned about the cost of medical care because they ultimately share in this cost, and they express this concern through the news media, health insurance companies, governmental agencies and various consumer-protection groups by questioning unnecessary surgery. This process is quite understandable from the consuming public's point of view. Of course the problem did not exist before insurance stepped in. **Go back to the days when patients paid their own way and—guess what—the public did not care.** Varicose surgery was not "unnecessary"; it was, from the public's and news media's point of view—invisible.

But look at the surgeon's position so far as varicose surgery is concerned. His patient asks him to remove her unsightly varicose veins. She claims they are causing her physical and psychological distress. Moreover, she has faithfully paid the premiums on her health insurance, which covers the cost of such surgery. What, then, should the surgeon do? That is the sixty-four dollar philosophical question—a question which I suspect lurks behind the whole fuzzy issue of unnecessary surgery.

While I totally reject the implication that callousness, incompetence, and irresponsibility are widespread among surgeons, I just as assuredly realize that some surgeons perform unnecessary surgery, that some surgeons are callous, and that incompetence has not been, and never will be, totally eliminated.

The best way to avoid unnecessary surgery is to place the decision in the hands of a trustworthy primary-care physician. If you have a physician who cares about your well-being, she is not going to permit unjustified surgery. In the first place, she will refer you to a surgeon only when, in her best judgment, an operation is necessary. The decision to operate is made by the surgeon but only with the full approval of your physician. Your physician knows your general condition best, she knows how much surgery you can physically tolerate and what the risks are and she is the one who must give the green light. The surgeon, on the other hand, renders his opinion about the feasibility of surgery and the type of operation best suited to resolve the problem.

A competent primary physician will choose a competent, trustworthy surgeon, a surgeon with a reputation among his colleagues for an honest and conservative approach. He is known for his caution. He is slow to recommend elective surgery and does so only after discussing it with the primary physician, and he fully explains the risks and goals to the patient.

You can see why it is important to choose a good primary physician. An irresponsible physician cares so little about her patients that she forces them to make their own choice of surgeons, never hinting that **certain surgeons are knife happy,**

out to make a quick buck by operating at the drop of a Blue Shield form. A good doctor cares enough about the well-being of her patients to steer them away from such notorious surgeons.

There are other ways to avoid unnecessary surgery. If you have any doubt about the integrity of your surgeon, get a second opinion when he recommends surgery. Most surgeons are honest in their surgical judgment, and do not savor putting people under the knife, risking lives just for the money. In obtaining a second opinion, you would have to be damned unlucky to run into two surgeons whose integrities were so low that they would collude in recommending an unnecessary operation.

When surgery is recommended, there are specific questions you should ask your surgeon: Why is the operation necessary? Are there drugs that could effect the same cure? What are the risks and do they outweigh the risks of not being operated on? Listen very carefully to his answers and watch his facial expression. If you detect doubt in his answers or in his facial expression, be cautious and **get a second opinion**. Cross-check the surgeon's answers with your primary physician. Ask whether the reasons the surgeon offers the surgery make sense to her. A good physician will have done all that groundwork for you, anyway. If she has any doubt about the intended surgery, she will be the first to talk to the surgeon about it.

The point I'm making is this: A good primary care physician is your most important asset in choosing a reputable surgeon. With a good physician as your advocate, everything else should follow automatically. That doesn't mean that you should sit back and do whatever she tells you without deciding for yourself. In the final analysis, it is you who are incurring the risk from a major operation; it behooves you to approach surgery intelligently and cautiously.

Paper credentials are of little value here. **Board certification is a requisite of the good surgeon but it is a minimum standard**. It guarantees neither the competency nor the integrity of a surgeon. I would never permit a non-board-certified surgeon to operate on me or a member of my family. But I would require far more information before allowing even a certified specialist to do the operation. I would rely very strongly on the advice and consent of a trustworthy primary physician.

Among the many types of surgery, several are commonly performed with meager justification. If your primary physician or surgeon recommends any of these, double-check to be sure they are necessary.

1. **Tonsillectomy:** There was a time, about seventy years ago, when tonsillectomy was recommended for almost every child. The slightest sore throat or infected ear prompted surgeons to recommend removal of the tonsils. Sometimes an entire family of children was lined up for routine tonsillectomies, almost as if fate had determined that at a given age the tonsils had to be removed. **My brother, my sister and myself underwent the operation on the same day and, bear in mind, my dad was a physician.**

This philosophy has changed radically over the past five decades. Very specific indications must exist to justify a tonsillectomy. If your physician recommends it, be cautious. Tonsillectomies are performed only in cases of recurrent ear infections where hearing loss occurs, cases with recurring, proven streptococcal infections, and where the massive size of the tonsils substantially impedes breathing. There is no way here to cover all the possible exceptions to these indications. You will have to depend on the joint recommendations of your primary physician and his surgical consultant. **Seek second opinions frequently**.

If you decide on tonsillectomy, a board certified specialist in ear, nose and throat surgery recommended by your primary physician should perform it. Some of the questions which you should ask this surgeon include the following:

In the case of children, what happens if we wait a few years? Is it not true that the tonsils will shrink during adolescence and solve the problem? Is there any danger in waiting for adolescence?

Can't infections, when due to streptococcus, be treated with penicillin? Will a tonsillectomy prevent recurrent infections?

2. **Hysterectomy:** This is often recommended, unnecessarily, when a woman is bleeding profusely or when she has back pain, ostensibly due to a large or backwardly displaced uterus. Cancer is a much more legitimate indication.

When your physician recommends hysterectomy, be certain to find out why. Cancer is an excellent reason. I have no hesitation in urging you to go along with a board-certified gynecologist who makes this recommendation. But excess bleeding and back pain are overused as reasons for recommending hysterectomies.

Bleeding often can be controlled with hormones, and back pain may have nothing to do with a backwardly displaced uterus. If your physician gives either of these reasons for performing a hysterectomy, be cautious. Ask the gynecologist if it is absolutely necessary to undergo surgery. Ask if hormones might not accomplish the same thing. Ask if he is certain your back pain is due to a displaced uterus. Go over his answers with your primary physician. Hysterectomy is a major operation. You should not take its risks lightly, however fashionable the operation may sound or however uncomfortable and distressed you may be. **Be cautious.**

3. **Varicose vein surgery**: Varicose veins are a common scourge of humanity. They appear as huge, ugly, snake-like purple swellings in the legs.

Removing these veins is a common operation done by board-certified general or vascular surgeons. Large, uncomfortable and unsightly veins can be stripped out of the legs by a competent surgeon or destroyed with laser treatments. Smaller, widespread purplish discolorations cannot easily be removed.

Varicose veins sometimes cause blood clots or phlebitis. They may also cause large, painful varicose ulcers near the ankles. Ulcers are due to invisible bleeding from swollen veins. The blood gathers under the skin and breaks down the nearby tissue, resulting in ulcers or open sores.

Varicose vein surgery is popular but frequently oversold. Women, quite naturally, do not like the appearance of varicose veins and often want them removed. Although the operation is a low risk procedure, it is attended by a couple of months of discomfort and a limitation on activities. **Furthermore, it cannot work miracles.** If you desire varicose vein surgery, discuss with a surgeon exactly what results he expects to obtain. Many people are disappointed because they expect far more than the operation can possibly deliver.

A good surgeon will examine your legs carefully and tell you what he can accomplish. Providing you understand the limitations of the operation and are willing to accept the risks and discomfort, I find nothing objectionable in this type of surgery. Be certain to discuss the many options now available for removal or ablation of varicose veins.

4. **Ruptured disc surgery**: An acutely ruptured disc, causing severe and disabling back pain, is a result of the upright position of the human animal and a common phenomenon. This problem can arise out of the blue and need not be associated with heavy lifting or other severe exertion. It is usually characterized by recurring back pain radiating down the buttocks, the back of the thigh and the lower legs.

If your physician suspects a ruptured disc and if the pain is severe and not relieved by bed rest or mild painkillers, he will recommend hospitalization. He may suggest a consultation with an orthopedic surgeon, a neurologist, or a neurosurgeon. Any of these specialists is competent to advise you on how to manage your disc problem.

Your physician should make every effort to treat your disc with rest, painkillers, muscle relaxants and traction. Frequently this will result in the complete relief of symptoms. Only under rare conditions should you consider surgery, and then only when evaluation proves that a disc is definitely ruptured. A knife-happy orthopedic surgeon or neurosurgeon can do a great deal of harm if the operation is performed unnecessarily. **Disc surgery is serious business.** Often injection with steroids can relieve the symptoms.

Discuss the situation with the surgeon. Ask him what he expects to accomplish, how sure he is that the operation will do the job, what the risks are, and what would happen if nonsurgical treatment were carried out for a week or two longer. Judge his reactions to these questions and discuss his answers with your primary physician. If you still have doubts, request a second opinion. A competent, self-confident surgeon will have no objection. But a surgeon who is incompetent will often blow his cool. Take this as a warning.

5. **Exploratory surgery**: Long-standing, unexplained, chronic abdominal pain sooner or later leads someone to suggest exploratory surgery. Typically, the patient has bounced around from one doctor to another seeking an explanation for his abdominal pain. X-rays, scans, blood tests and other special procedures have failed to uncover the cause. Some doctors have told him to "live with the pain"; others have blamed it on his nerves, and still others have given the pain a fancy label such as "spastic colitis" or said that it comes from an "irritable colon,"

terms which mean nothing but cover the doctor's ignorance by appearing to **label the disease**.

Then some doctor recommends an exploratory operation. The patient has tried drugs, psychological counseling and exercise programs. All have failed—the patient still suffers unremitting, disabling pain. Depressed, confused about modern medicine's inability to ferret out its cause, and exasperated by the futility of each diagnostic adventure, the patient is receptive to the suggestion that an exploratory operation might solve the problem. The unethical surgeon, opportunist that he always is, looks for this type of patient, and offers him the hope, often unfounded, that surgery may be the answer.

Unfortunately the odds against surgery relieving chronic abdominal pain are overwhelming. Modern X-ray, cat scans, MRIs and other diagnostic testing have rendered exploratory operations almost obsolete. In the vast majority of cases, such an exploration not only fails to uncover the cause of the pain, but compounds the problem by adding the risk and discomfort of the operation and the possibility that subsequent surgical adhesions will lead to more trouble later.

If your surgeon suggests exploratory surgery, **be circumspect**. Discuss it with your primary physician and the surgeon. Ask what the odds are of such surgery finding anything that hasn't already been uncovered by diagnostic evaluations. Ask about the risks, the possibility that you will be worse off. Ask about the possibility of managing the problem with medication, dietary regimen or just plain **tincture of time**. Do not overlook the possibility that the problem may be more emotional than organic. When this is the case, a little insight may permit you to live with the pain more comfortably.

In the end, you'll have to trust the wisdom and judgment of your primary physician and your own ability to evaluate the integrity of the surgeon. **Always request a second surgical opinion before undergoing an exploratory operation**.

At times you will have no choice. As long as you go into this operation as a last resort I have no objection. I perform this operation very rarely indeed and always tell my patients that there is less that a five percent chance that I will find a correctible problem. I have found that a thorough discussion of the odds and a totally honest approach at least makes the patient feel, if the operation is unsuccessful, that no stone was left unturned and that the operation was worth the risk as a last resort.

I have described these particular operations because they are frequently performed and involve some general principles that you can apply to any operation. Caution and circumspection are the watchwords whenever surgery is recommended. **In spite of modern techniques, major surgery still has its risks.**

The following three cases illustrate the problems of surgical judgment and philosophy. They show why you should question your surgeon about any proposed major surgery and why you should get a second opinion.

The first patient, a 50 year old, came to me complaining of vague abdominal pain of several months duration, made worse by eating heavy foods. Testing revealed gallstones. It was my opinion that the pain was due to these gallstones and that the gall bladder should be removed. The patient quizzed me at length about the indications for surgery, what the operation was designed to accomplish, whether any form of medical therapy would do the same job, what the risks would be if he decided against surgery, and so on.

I told him that the ideal treatment for his gallstones was to have his gall bladder removed and that there was no effective substitute. I informed him that if he chose not to have the surgery he should remain on a low-fat diet to minimize his discomfort, although he would probably continue to have some pain. I told him there was a small chance that he would develop serious problems, namely, an acute attack of gall bladder disease or, worse, a blockage of his bile ducts from the stones. He wanted to know what the chances were of such a serious complication occurring if he chose not to have the operation. I told him that it was impossible to say but there was a fair chance that serious trouble would set in eventually.

He decided against the operation because of an overriding fear of surgery in spite of the low complications from laparoscopic surgery. I did not think it fair to push him. I told him to contact me at the first sign of any worsening of the symptoms and that I wanted to check him every six months to be certain nothing was going on insidiously. He agreed and I have examined him for seven years. He has developed no signs of serious trouble. He lucked out but he still kids me about "unnecessary surgery."

Well, is it? That depends on the individual case and how things happen to work out. I believe my recommendation was sound. It was based on the likelihood that, sooner or later, many such patients have serious trouble with gallstones. His pain only occurs with dietary indiscretions. He suffers no serious side effects and may continue this way indefinitely. **Looked at from his point of view, surgery was not really necessary**. My point: some operations are more necessary than others.

Pin down the surgeon as to the necessity of surgery when he recommends it. Find out just what the consequences may be if you choose not to follow the surgeon's advice. It is your body and you alone incur the risks either way.

The second patient, 80, had cancer of the rectum. The surgeon recommended an extensive operation which would have required removal of the rectum and creation of a permanent colostomy. The patient's granddaughter felt that her grandfather, who was failing rapidly from old age and senility, wouldn't be able to manage a colostomy even if he did survive the formidable operative procedure. She asked if surgery were absolutely necessary, and he replied that there was no other form of treatment that could effectively remove the cancer and prevent its recurrence.

Not satisfied, she sought the opinion of a second surgeon. He agreed with the diagnosis and also agreed that only surgery could cure the cancer. However, he recognized the patient's advanced age and senility and said that he could also perform a very minor operation which would consist of burning out the tumor without removing the rectum or fashioning a colostomy. He said this would not cure the disease but would relieve the symptoms for, perhaps, several months. The granddaughter instinctively felt that this was the better choice. She gave her approval and the operation was carried out successfully. The patient lived for about a year and died of a heart attack with no recurrence of the cancer. He remained in control of his bowels and, of course, did not suffer the inconvenience of a permanent colostomy.

This is a good illustration of the value of a second opinion. Both surgeons arrived at the same diagnosis and both recommended major surgery and a colostomy as the only effective treatment. However, the second surgeon had a better grasp of the situation: **the patient's short life expectancy**, the difficulty he would have managing his colostomy and the anxieties of the granddaughter, who instinctively felt that the least done the better.

By conferring with a second surgeon, the granddaughter was better able to reconcile her perception of the reality of the situation with the treatment.

Was the first surgeon remiss in his responsibility in recommending unnecessary surgery? I do not think so. This was a case of a different philosophical outlook on the part of the two surgeons.

The third patient, 79, had a small groin hernia. It was not causing him any difficulty but he was anxious to find out if it was dangerous. The surgeon recommended an operation because he felt that the hernia would eventually enlarge and cause difficulty. There was always the chance that it would strangulate—a very serious problem.

The patient decided to get a second opinion and received an entirely different recommendation. He was told that surgery was not necessary. The second surgeon felt that, since the patient was 79 and very sedentary, it was unlikely that the hernia would grow significantly. At any rate, he would check it every six months and alter his opinion in favor of surgery if he noted any significant growth rate. As for strangulation, he agreed that it was a possibility, but a slim one in view of the small size and type of hernia. If the patient was cautious and called at the first sign of local pain over the hernia, the surgeon could operate, preventing any trouble.

The patient was anxious about strangulation. He went back to the first surgeon and underwent the operation and did quite well, secure that the danger had been removed.

Who was right? **Everybody!** The first surgeon was correct in warning the patient about the danger of strangulation. The patient was wise in seeking a second opinion and, when he continued to feel anxious, having the operation anyway. The second surgeon was also correct in playing down the chance of strangulation, and suggesting as an alternative that the patient be alert for local groin pain. He also recommended a six-month check-up.

Am I saying that the operation was both necessary and unnecessary? It's all relative to the situation. Some operations, like an appendectomy for a ruptured appendix, are categorically necessary. There can be no two ways about it. Other operations, like the removal of the rectum for cancer, often depend on the patient's life expectancy, age, senility, and other medical problems. Still others, like the hernia repair in the 79-year-old man, can be managed either way with perfect justification. After all, it is the patient who is incurring all the risks and he alone must weigh the judgments of his physicians.

A second opinion is designed not so much to check on a surgeon's integrity or competency as it is to observe how the judgment and philosophy of one surgeon differs from those of another. By bouncing the same questions off two surgeons, you will get an idea of the possible advantages and disadvantages of surgery from different points of view. By comparing these opinions with the recommendation of your personal physician, you will be able to judge the wisdom of the proposed surgery.

How do you go about getting a second opinion? Will the first surgeon be upset? Be frank about the whole thing. Tell the first surgeon that you would feel better with a second, independent opinion. If he is competent and self-confident, he is unlikely to object. He would probably do the same thing if another surgeon recommended surgery for him and he wasn't sure of the wisdom of the operation. Be sure to make the second opinion an independent one, not based on a referral from the first surgeon.

If you get a second opinion and decide to go along with it, let the first surgeon know, simply as a matter of courtesy. But it is not necessary, and if you feel uneasy about it, you don't have to. Let your primary physician know what you decide so she can discuss your case with the second surgeon.

Time Out!

By now I think you get the point that your primary care physician is your most important bodyguard against any mistakes in treatment, be it medical or surgical.

Further, as I have emphasized again and again throughout this little book, second and third opinions are vital for you and offer yet again a blockage against wrong therapy.

I hope by now that your skepticism about YOU being the most important judge of the good doctor is beginning to make sense to you. Can you imagine any "quality assurance" or "quality improvement" team or government agency being able to figure out all the subtleties I have brought to your attention thus far in this book?

Chapter 16: The Doctor as a Confidant

"too hot to handle?"

Chapter summary: This chapter starts by describing several "doctor" images used by television "soap operas" over the years, what they were trying to do and why most of them failed except for Marcus Welby. He was, as I said earlier, a *confidant* of the patient and I go on to describe why this image attracted viewers far more than other TV doctor "heroes." If you are looking for a confidant, and I will define that term, then there are several important things you must know about your choice of doctors.

Literature gives us many models of the American physician but it has taken the power of television to distill these mythologies and project them, embellished and over-dramatized, into tangible personalities.

First, there was Dr. Kildare: young, bright and inexperienced, but extremely eager to learn from his older mentor, Dr. Gillespie. He was idealistic but not naive. He believed in social justice and egalitarianism and was thrilled with each new adventure in healing and solace. Kildare had his moment in the sun, but he didn't quite wash with the American people. He did better with the reading public and moviegoers. Overexposed on television, his star rapidly faded. **What was wrong with Kildare? He was simply unreal**. Too clean-cut, too youthful in his ideals, he lacked the kind of bedrock confidence desired by the average American.

Then came Ben Casey, almost the opposite of calm, clean-cut Kildare. He was harsh, judgmental, extremely well trained in modern medical techniques and, like Kildare, a great egalitarian. He didn't make it either. His popularity peaked rapidly. **There was something too coarse about Ben Casey.** Perhaps it was his appearance or his manners, but I suspect it was the lack of gentility people expect of physicians.

Star Trek, that space travel fantasy, gave us "Bones," a nonperson of a physician famous for his near-perfect command of the technology of diagnosis and healing. The sick spaceman was placed in a formidable-looking diagnostic chamber, lights blinked, and a computer printed out the diagnosis and prescribed treatment. Bones did nothing but act as the interpreter between machine and patient. **Television had struck on the mythology of a supertechnician, an infallible combination of brains and machine but no soul**. Few people warmed to this transistorized medico and Bones took a back seat in *Star Trek*.

The granddaddy of the television physicians was Marcus Welby. For several years, in the heyday of black and white television, twenty million people remained glued to their television screens, fascinated and charmed by this grey-haired, middle-aged family physician. What was Welby's attraction? What chord did he touch that made him a near permanent television fixture in the medical personalities?

The writers and producers had discovered what people were looking for in a physician. They distilled and personalized it and came up with Marcus Welby—a role containing characteristics of earlier television medical heroes. There was the idealism of Kildare, the justice and drive of Casey and the supreme technical skill of Star Trek's Bones. But tying all these characteristics together was a new element—**a humanism which permitted Welby to be a warm confidant to all his patients.**

Now there's nothing wrong with any of these famous models. What is important is what you expect in a physician. If you are looking for the ultimate, infallible, nonperson technician, such as Bones, you'll never be satisfied with a hard-hitting, emotional Ben Casey. If Kildare's youth and adventurism turn you on, you won't be satisfied with Marcus Welby, no matter how bedrock, charming, and fatherly.

Half the dissatisfaction with doctors today is due to this confusion of images. People who stared at Welby for years, with his total commitment to his patients and their tragedies, his disinterest in money, his expertise in many fields of medicine, are in for a shock when they bump into a real physician who expects to be paid for his work and doesn't have all the answers.

What image you have of your doctor and what kind of relationship you want to have with him or her are important factors in your choice. If you're looking for a confidant, be sure you have a doctor who is willing to discuss matters outside medicine. If he freezes the moment you bring up a marital problem, for example, then you've got the wrong doctor. A good doctor, a confidant, may be the best person to talk to when domestic and psychological problems seem to overwhelm you.

If your doctor is to be your confidant, you must be able to trust him with confidential information. He must be frank with you without being a moralist. He must have a balanced, open-minded view and be willing to take the time to talk to you. If he's too busy to handle these kinds of problems, re-think your choice. He may not be the doctor for you.

A confidant, like a friend, is concerned about you and cares about you. Some problems require the support and advice of a friend. Others can destroy that friendship. **Problems which are too hot for a friend to handle should be placed in the hands of a confidant**. A trusting, caring, personal physician may be just what you need.

Time Out!

Wouldn't it be so much better and more professional to place confidential information and thoughts in the hand of a counselor or psychologist? Why use an expensive, technique-oriented physician for this type of bruising information?

It really depends on a number of factors. To begin with, it may be that a counselor is better for your problem. Where do you begin to sort this out?

At times your medical problems may be somewhat responsible for your psychological problems and the primary care physician is a good place to start. He or she may sense better than a counselor when the problem is medical and when it is truly psychological or sociological.

If you do not already have a counselor I would strongly suggest you begin by discussing these problems with your physician provided you see him as a confidant. If he feels the problem is best handled by a counselor or a psychologist he will be the best source of referral for you.

Chapter 17: What You Should Know About Drugs

"more than a grain of salt"

Chapter summary: Drugs are a vital part of medical care, are used by every physician and also are responsible for serious illness, even death, far more often than people or most physicians really know. There are hundreds upon hundreds of drugs; they come and go. There are incompatible drugs, drugs with fatal side effects, drugs often prescribed too hastily. Here I define the problem, then list ten safety steps which you must apply to each drug before taking it, and add some very important questions to ask the doctor before taking the drugs. The doctor's answers go a long way to letting you know whether you have chosen a good doctor.

No medicine is entirely safe. Each pill you swallow alters the physiology of your body and sets in motion a new sequence of events not entirely predictable even by the most astute physician. Modern drugs are extremely powerful and must be taken with great care and under constant supervision.

Drug-induced illness is reaching epidemic proportions. A large percentage of hospital admissions are due to complications from prescription drugs. The variety of complications and catastrophes described in many studies of drug-induced illnesses are too numerous to list. Studies of hospitalized patients have shown a ten to eighteen percent incidence of adverse drug reactions with a fatality rate as high as thirteen percent. These adverse reactions are occurring right under the noses of doctors and nurses in spite of their constant surveillance.

A substantial part of doctoring consists of the prudent and timely prescription of strong drugs to alter the course of disease in a beneficial way. You can get a good idea about how competent your doctor is by observing how he handles drugs and explains their dangers to you. **A good doctor has a healthy respect for drugs.** It is most important that he transmit that respect to you. This chapter won't make you a drug expert and it cannot be used as a guide to the safe use of drugs. Its purpose is to make you aware of some of the basic problems of using prescription drugs so you can judge how well your physician handles the matter.

The dimensions of the problem have only recently come to the attention of the medical profession. Stimulated by the Thalidomide tragedy of the 1960s, registries of adverse drug reactions have cropped up as physicians and pharmacists document and analyze adverse reactions.

You may wonder how all this can happen in this day of modern quality control. Indeed a whole science of drug-induced diseases exists. The number of federal, state, and private agencies that concern themselves with drug hazards testifies to the breadth and depth of the problem. The research, development, and final marketing of a new drug is one of the most carefully monitored practices in existence today. Ethical drug houses can ill afford a repeat of the Thalidomide tragedy. And yet, tragedies and oversights still occur.

The Food and Drug Administration (FDA) exerts an extremely tight monitoring control over the development and marketing of drugs. It evaluates short- and long-term effects of new medications and controls the quality of manufacturing and packaging of standard drugs. **While the FDA is sometimes accused of undue harassment, it has discharged its responsibilities with a high degree of professionalism and competency over the years.**

The American Medical Association's Council on Drugs, from its inception in 1905, has aided practicing physicians by providing up-to-date information on the safety and efficacy of drug products. The members of this council are among the most authoritative physicians in the field of drug research and therapy.

The Council maintains a constant watch over drug hazards and is in continuous communication with AMA physicians.

Modern drugs are effective precisely because they alter the body's chemistry, which is also what makes them so potentially dangerous. Quality control, animal experimentation and strict regulation by various agencies eliminate some of the problems but they have no effect on physicians who prescribe these drugs dangerously or on patients who use them unintelligently. **The final and most important quality control team is your doctor and yourself.**

The physician is the last monitor of a drug's use and quality control. Because he is responsible for the safety of his patient, he must weigh the risks of therapy against the risks of untreated disease. He must weigh one therapeutic method against another, monitor the effects of a drug or combination of drugs on his patient and on the disease, be alert for adverse drug reactions and maintain an expertise that enables him to distinguish the symptoms of drug reaction from symptoms of the disease itself. **Finally he must transmit a sense of this responsibility to his patients by explaining the hazards of drugs and educating them about precautions to be taken in their use.**

Education about drug hazards should begin with your physician informing you of the name and nature of the drug you are to take. It is amazing how many patients are unaware of these facts. I have frequently heard a patient say, "I am taking a little pink, round pill for my heart and two water pills for my excess fluid." That is the sum of his knowledge. The unwillingness of many physicians to label each prescription with the name of the drug is a survival from an earlier tradition that considered it unwise to tell patients about their disease or its treatment. It was feared that informed patients would develop a morbid curiosity so that it was the physician's duty to protect his patients from the unsettling influence of too much knowledge.

In simpler times this might have been a prudent policy. Families did not move around much and the one family doctor knew his patients well, often for a lifetime, and knew everything they had in their medicine cabinets. Nor were the drugs in his black bag as powerful as they are today. While they failed to do much good, they probably did little harm.

Things are different today. Families change doctors frequently through either choice or relocation. Often two or three specialists are prescribing simultaneously for one patient; each may be unaware of the full spectrum of drugs the patient is taking. As a result, drug incompatibilities pose hazards to patients ignorant of the vagaries of pharmacology. Certain drugs may antagonize or neutralize each other's effects; worse, two drugs may amplify each other's effects, resulting in an unexpected and dangerous overreaction.

Patients assume that the drug companies, the government and their physicians will see to it that no harm comes to them from the medicines they take. This is a dangerous assumption. While inherent hazards of new drugs are carefully screened, it is essential that the patient, with her individual psychological and physiological variables, take the pill (alone or in combination with others) at the right time and under the right circumstances. She must not take the wrong pill, the wrong number of pills or the wrong combination of pills. She must not take pills that have lost their potency, pills prescribed for illnesses in the past, or pills that are incompatible with other pills. Some pills can be taken at any time while others must not be taken while driving or during other hazardous activities. Many pills cause idiosyncratic or unpredictable symptoms. Some are unsafe during pregnancy; others are not. Some pills cause exactly the opposite effect they are intended to cause in certain people.

The patient bears a responsibility to herself to understand the drugs she consumes. No medicine is entirely safe. Quality control and safety begin with the drug house responsible for marketing of the pill and end with the patient who administers the drug. The pitfalls and hazards of self-medication without knowledge of the name and effect of the drug are incalculable. Mix ups in dosages, incompatible drugs, failure to understand early warning signs of complications, all can be diminished or eliminated by educating patients about drug hazards. **The patient is the last controlling agent before the pill hits the bloodstream.**

The basic safety rules for the taking of pills are as follows:

1. **Avoid using pills, capsules, and other forms of medicine if at all possible**.
    a. No drug is entirely safe.

b. Too often pills are used where diet, exercise, and other general good health measures would safely accomplish much more.

2. Do not take a pill if you don't know its name, its nature and the effect it will have on you.

a. Insist that your physician or pharmacist label the prescription.

b. Ask your doctor about the drug. Ask him what it is for, how it works, what are its side effects and dangers. You will be surprised how gratified he will be that you are sincerely interested and knowledgeable enough to ask intelligent questions.

c. Avoid over-the-counter medications as much as possible, unless you have discussed their value and safety with your doctor.

d. Throw away all unlabeled pills no matter how good your memory is.

3. Never restart a pill you have been off for some time with the mistaken assumption that, "I've got the same symptoms; must be the same trouble; why bother calling the doctor?"

a. You may be wrong about the diagnosis.

b. You may be on another pill, which is incompatible with the new pill.

4. Never take a pill prescribed for a friend, neighbor, or relative on the mistaken assumption that you've "got the same symptoms; must be the same illness."

a. You may be wrong about the similarity of symptoms.

b. Your body may not tolerate the same pill.

c. Your neighbor's doctor may be wrong.

d. If you are concerned enough to start pills, consult your doctor about your illness.

5. Never take a pill other than on the advice of a trusted physician.

6. **If you have more than one pill, particularly from more than one doctor, review their use and continued indications with your family doctor. Be wary of drug combinations.**

7. **Review your medical inventory or medicine cabinet periodically.**
   - **a.** Throw away all unlabeled pills.
   - **b.** Throw away all labeled pills prescribed for a former illness which you do not now have.
   - **c.** Throw away all pills over a year old, as they may have deteriorated.
   - **d.** Keep a checklist of all your medications and label the number of pills left in each bottle periodically. This information may be very useful if a child accidentally swallows the remaining pills.

8. **Know as much as you can about your past illnesses and reactions to medications. When placed on a new pill, review these illnesses and reactions with your physician.**

9. **Report to your physician any symptoms beginning after the taking of the medication. These symptoms may be due to the pill you are taking rather than to the disease for which you are being treated.**

10. **Most importantly, develop a high respect for all medicines and encourage your children to do likewise.**

. If you wish to know more about the drugs you are taking, consult the librarian at your local hospital. Unless you have a background in pharmacology, however, I think you'd best satisfy your curiosity by a thorough discussion with your physician. A good doctor, one who cares about you as a person, will make time for such discussions. He will want you to be satisfied about the drug he is asking you to take. Beware of the doctor who puts you down with a gentle smile and the glib remark: "Now don't be worried. Just take the pill I've prescribed and everything will be fine."

Let's suppose you've been handed a prescription for a drug and you haven't chosen to ask anything about the drug. What is the obligation of your physician under these circumstances? It is his duty to tell you the name and nature of the drug, its purpose, its side effects and complications, the symptoms of these side effects and complications, and whether it is incompatible with any other drug you might be taking. Furthermore, he must ask you for a detailed drug history to ascertain if you have ever taken this or similar drugs and, if so, whether you have ever had any complications.

1. **Use this checklist to judge how well your physician handles the hazards of prescription drugs:**

2. **How well does your physician educate you about the drugs he has prescribed?**
3. **Does he label each prescription and tell you the name and nature of the drug?**
4. **Does he tell you what the drug is for and how it works?**
5. **Does he alert you to the side effects of the drug?**
6. **Does he warn you about the drug's potential complications and what symptoms you should look for?**
7. **Does he tell you what drugs are incompatible with the drug you are about to take?**
8. **To put it in a nutshell: Since drugs are so hazardous, has your physician made a reasonable effort to warn you of this?**

Time Out!

If physicians make mistake after mistake about the safety and dangers of drugs, how am I to know more than they do about the risks?

So argues the reasonable patient, and why not? How are you able to judge what is a dangerous drug or combination of dangerous drugs? Isn't this really the job of the primary care physician?

Yes of course, providing your physician is cautious and concerned about your well-being, provided he or she is a good doctor. That is the whole point of this book. How are you to know, at first, who is the good doctor?

You cannot! It will take more than a few visits to the doctor you have initially chosen and then you must apply every principle laid down in this book. Review each chapter from time to time. Like learning to ride a bicycle, it tasks practice, but you can get there if you make the effort.

Chapter 18: How to Get the Most Out of a Visit to Your Doctor

"like herding cats"

Chapter summary: This is a key chapter in this day of managed care in which a doctor is compelled to watch the clock and limit your visit. This chapter attempts two things: 1. To help you organize your symptoms so that you can present your case very efficiently and yet thoroughly to the doctor and 2. To teach you how to manage your doctor and make demands for necessary care when he or she is trying to ration that care. **There are some simple rules to this game and I will attempt to make you the winner every time.**

Today's physician is extremely short on time. It is unlikely that your visits have given you a comprehensive picture of your health needs. What do you know about the total state of your health? What do you know about the condition of your organ systems? What do you know about the adequacy of your own health practices? Do you have a prognosis for a healthy future without disability?

If you are a woman of 35, with children, you probably visited your pediatrician twice last year, your gynecologist once, and your internist once or twice. You spent hours in waiting rooms and a good deal of money for babysitting, transportation and other expenses. If you are a woman over 60, you saw your physician approximately six times for problems such as persistent headaches, vaginal discharge, and prolonged stomach pains. Between her fees, lab work, and X-rays, you paid a great deal of money for this care.

After all of these visits and expenses, what do you know about your total health? Probably not as much as you would like. **One way to get at this problem is to prepare yourself for each visit to your physician**.

Step 1: Plan the right type of visit.

Arrange a full visit with your doctor by telling her secretary that you wish a complete checkup and you wish to discuss fully the status of your health. The average office visit lasts ten minutes—totally inadequate for a comprehensive examination. If you show up for a routine appointment, your physician will listen to your complaints and treat the individual symptoms. This may solve your immediate problem but it is inadequate in terms of your total health needs. Far better to wait longer and arrange for a **comprehensive health examination**. Beware if the secretary has a hesitant gulp in her voice when you ask for this type of visit.

Step 2: Organize your symptoms

Organize your symptoms and **arrive at one or more clearly defined chief complaints**. A chief complaint represents a main symptom or cluster of symptoms which makes you seek medical attention. If you have no symptoms and are going for a general checkup, then there is no need to pursue this step any further. More often, however, there are immediate symptoms which prompt a patient to make an appointment and it is these symptoms that you should work out in detail before you visit your doctor.

Step 3: Think about your symptoms

Develop your chief complaint by asking yourself a series of relevant questions. For example, if your complaint is a nagging cough, you might ask yourself: "How long have I had the cough? Is it getting worse? Is the cough associated with the production of sputum and, if so, has there ever been any blood mixed with this sputum? Do I have any shortness of breath or chest pain associated with this cough? How many cigarettes do I smoke a day?"

Another example is abdominal pain: "In what part of my abdomen is this pain located? Does it radiate to any other part of my abdomen? Is the pain worse before or after meals? Is it relieved by a bowel movement? Have I had any associated vomiting or intolerance to certain foods?"

There is no set pattern to these questions. **The important thing is to examine your complaints in detail so that you can organize and present them to your physician**. Many of the questions which she will ask will help you analyze your symptoms further. You don't have to think of all the possible questions that can be asked. That is her job.

By thinking about your complaint and analyzing its symptoms, you will give your doctor a better insight into the possible causes of your ailment. Nothing is more distressing to a busy physician than to have a patient who cannot describe his symptoms. He rambles on, unable to tell how long he has had the symptoms, whether they are better or worse than previously, worse during the day or at night, or associated with meals, exertion, work or exercise.

A physician is more apt to be interested in your complaint if she senses that you are. I have frequently interviewed patients who appeared to be so blasé about their complaints that I wondered why they have come in the first place.

Step 4. Be brief, relevant, but thorough

Be brief and relevant in describing your complaints and in answering your doctor's questions. Time is limited; use it most effectively.

The following example from my office records is of a woman who complained of shoulder pain. Notice her garrulousness and how her irrelevancies confuse the issue and exasperate the doctor.

Doctor: What seems to be bothering you today, Mrs. L.?

Mrs. L: Well, I haven't been feeling too well lately, Doctor. It's this pain I'm having.

Doctor: Where is the pain, Mrs. L.?

Mrs. L.: Well, it's pretty hard to describe. It seems to be located somewhere here (pointing to her shoulder).

Doctor: How long have you had the pain, Mrs. L.?

Mrs. L.: Well, I was on my way to the supermarket about two weeks ago ... no, let me see, it probably was about three weeks ago. I had just finished my shopping and was on my way out to the car to bring the food to my niece's house at her summer camp…

Doctor: (interrupting) Were you lifting a heavy package at the time the pain began?

Mrs. L: As I said, I was on my way to my niece's...blah… blah… blah…

Step 5: Define your goals for the visit

Be clear about your goals for each visit. The tragedy of most visits to the doctor is that the patient's goals are too narrow. The patient wishes to have his complaints evaluated, diagnosed and treated. He is unaware of the more important general goals, namely, an evaluation of the total status of his health and health practices, a prognosis and advice. While it is understandable that patients want to have their complaints—a nagging headache or sore throat—taken care of, it is important that they realize that far more serious health problems may be lurking in the background.

How tragic to have a 40 year-old woman seen three times by her physician for a sore throat without anyone discovering that a small detectable breast cancer is beginning to develop. For want of a proper breast examination, her cancer could develop beyond the curable phase under the physician's eyes.

In a comprehensive visit to your physician the following goals are a minimum:

1. An evaluation of your chief complaint or complaints.

2. A general discussion of your current total health status.

3. A general discussion of your current health practices.

4. Your prognosis as far as can be developed for future health and well-being.

5. Your particular health needs, if any.

Step 6: Know your past medical history.

Your past history is always relevant and should be included in your discussion with your physician. The most important parts of your history include:

1. Previous major surgery.
2. Previous hospitalization for major illnesses.
3. Previous use of drugs for whatever illness.
4. Any drug allergies in the past.

Spend more time reviewing your past history before visiting your doctor. Write down, in chronological order, all your previous illnesses, hospitalizations and operations, along with the treatment, complications, and results. This will not only save your doctor time but it will let her know that you are concerned about your health. Such a list will look something like this:

Mary J., age 71

1947: Hospitalized and had tonsils out—no problems.

1951: Discovered to have high blood pressure, placed on medication—discontinued on my own two years later; no follow-up exams.

1957: Hepatitis: treated at home for two weeks; no further problems.

1960: Underwent removal of gall bladder; developed pneumonia after surgery; stayed in hospital ten days; also told I had mild diabetes.

Step 7: Make a list of the drugs you are taking

Your medication history is extremely important. Be certain you know the names of pills you are taking. Check with your pharmacist before going to the doctor. If this is not possible, bring the pills and their prescription numbers, and the doctor or his secretary will check them out.

Nothing is more disconcerting than to have a patient come in with a pocketbook full of half-filled bottles of pills in various colors, sizes and shapes, with no labels to indicate what they are, how frequently you have been taking them, or how long. **Some patients are walking medicine cabinets with absolutely no understanding of the nature of their medications.** It's not just the elderly; patients of all ages are ignorant of drug therapy. It is incredible that educated and informed adults, conscious of things such as spoilage of their ecology, the latest fad in diets, and the remotest hazards of certain foods, will swallow all manner of pills on direction of their physician without having the foggiest idea of what they are or what side effect they may produce.

Step 8: Know your family history

Family history is important to your physician. If your immediate parents, brothers, sisters or children suffer from chronic disease such as high blood pressure, tuberculosis, malignancy, diabetes, arthritis, allergies, emphysema, vascular disease, or kidney disease, your doctor will want to know. It may have a bearing on the state of your health. Make a list of such family illnesses.

Step 9: Know your health habits

You should know your dietary history, work habits, exercise and relaxation patterns, and habits with respect to alcohol and nicotine. Write these down and don't be afraid to read from your notes or give them to your doctor. **Written notes and other signs of an organized patient will always capture the attention of the physician and gain you more time.**

In summary, to get the most out of your visit, arrange the right type of appointment, spend a good deal of time investigating and organizing your symptoms, make a list of your past medical problems and family history. Be aware of your health practices in detail. Do not withhold any information. Ask your physician all the questions you think are necessary and don't leave his office until you have a comprehensive understanding of your present health status. Bear in mind that your good health is largely a function of how well you are able to comply with your physician's recommendations and admonitions.

Physicians respond to a well-organized patient's presentation. They are like cats but can be herded.

Time Out!

Are you trying to tell me that my little notes about my past or family history have any real value in this day of high tech scans, MRIs and fancy genetic testing?

Does it really benefit me to walk in with a list of pills I am taking? Isn't this old fashioned? Doesn't the doctor just order a bunch of fancy tests and the diagnosis pops out?

Yes, yes, no, no!

Your history of your problem, believe it or not, is far more important in the diagnostic process than most tests a doctor can order. That may sound hard to believe, but you must trust me in this matter. I have spent fifteen years with second-year medical students at a prominent Boston medical school, training them in physical diagnosis, the beginning of the diagnostic process. The whole point of this course is to emphasize to these students how critical the taking of a proper history is from the patient. A full and accurate diagnosis cannot be made with fancy technology except for acute emergency room trauma problems. **The key to a good diagnosis is what the patient tells you about his problem.**

Chapter 19: Underdoctoring and Overdoctoring

"disease vs. dis-ease"

Chapter summary: The definition and explanation of the terms "under-" and "over-" doctoring explain vividly what it is all about, especially in this period of managed care. You must learn all you can about the two bad forms of medical care, and compel your doctor to avoid both. If he fails, you must come to recognize that you have not made a good choice of doctors and it is time to move on.

Underdoctoring

How much "doctoring" should you expect? How much do you need? Unfortunately, what you need and what you expect or demand aren't always the same.

People seem to think they are not getting enough doctoring unless a whole battery of fancy and intricate blood tests and X-rays are performed ritually every year or so. This, the so-called executive physical, was oversold to the public and to the medical profession by an opportunistic medical-industrial complex in the 1950s and 1960s.

Underdoctoring is not the failure to perform a lot of tests. Nor is it a failure to prescribe a lot of drugs, exotic diets or ritualized exercise programs. It is a failure on the part of your doctor to teach you the art of healthy living when you are well and to work hard to uncover disease when you are ill. It is an inability or unwillingness on your doctor's part to view you and your family as his total medical responsibility, in health and in sickness, while you live, and as you die.

Underdoctoring is a failure of a doctor's will far more often than his intellect. You can sense and feel it in a thousand different ways. Concern, hard work, thoroughness, follow-through, caring, availability, affability, teaching, sympathizing, understanding—these are what you must look for in your doctor. These are the ingredients that are missing in underdoctoring, not a lot of tests and procedures.

Consider your doctor's attitude before you worry about his aptitude. Observe the little things he does, not the big words he uses. The tests he orders are not half as important as your test of how much he cares about you. Underdoctoring exists when diseases are discovered and treated in a vacuum, disconnected from the patient and unrelated to his loved ones.

Underdoctoring exists when your doctor removes a wart from your arm because you requested it and fails to remove that pack of cigarettes from your pocket or at least talk it over with you. Underdoctoring occurs when your doctor observes that your blood pressure has increased but fails to note that your waistline has also. The modern physician gets angry with the lab for being late with your blood-test report. The old-time doctor got angry with his patient for pushing too hard or drinking too much.

The authoritarian who browbeats you because he cares may not be such a bad doctor after all. You can always fire him! **You have been underdoctored when your prudent, modern doctor coddles you more than he cajoles you**. Caring sometimes means cussing and there is something to be said for irascibility at times.

Underdoctoring is a vacuous feeling you get that your doctor is a professional entity who works over in "that medical office building"; that, for a fee and by appointment, he can be turned on to your medical problem, possibly solving it with fancy tests and powerful drugs; that, barring an emergency, when his shades go down and his lights go out, so goes his relationship with you. **He wraps up his care in discrete packages and delivers it with skill "by appointment only." That is the essence of underdoctoring.**

Overdoctoring

Mr. Suburbanite, an informed, haughty senior executive, knows better than most about good medical care. On schedule and without fail, faithfully and unquestioning, he enters the Mecca of Medicine, the high-powered medical-school clinic, and exposes his body to an army of technicians, nurses and specialists. Questions are asked, exams are done, and blood is drawn. An extraordinary series of X-rays and special procedures are brought to bear on his symptom-free, healthy body, which turn out to be normal, as expected.

He is given a full report of his normalcy and told to report again next year. **This is the executive physical examination, the ultimate in overdoctoring**.

An 89 year-old woman sustained a painful fractured hip and is operated on successfully. The wound heals and she should be able to return home. Now starts the overdoctoring.

Somebody discovers that her blood pressure is low and a series of tests is set in motion. Somebody else discovers a spot on her lung, and another specialist imposes on her sanity and sanctity to "make sure it isn't cancer," as if it really mattered.

What about her newly discovered heart murmur? Call in the cardiologist, of course; mustn't miss a weakened heart valve. There's an abnormality in her urine! Could it be a failing kidney? Can't find out without a urologist who does twelve more tests.

On and on it goes. This 89 year-old woman will spend four weeks in the hospital and get to know six specialists, not well, only by name and specialty. They come and go too fast for her to recall. **This is also overdoctoring.**

Technology is neutral. It can be used or abused, applied or misapplied. It all depends on the doctor's wisdom and his sense of proportion and disproportion.

Overdoctoring is an ever-present temptation. It is legally and professionally safer and more lucrative to overtest and overtreat. It is easier to take a test than to talk to a patient and examine him, applying technology with discrimination.

Overdoctoring is part of our technological imperative, an obsession to use every trick available so that disease will not happen and death will be denied. But unless people can be taught to take care of their bodies and minds, technology comes to naught and overdoctoring ironically turns into underdoctoring. We have come full circle.

Overdoctoring and underdoctoring are intimately related. They are different facets of the same problem—both part of the profession's failure to see the humanity of patients, to balance teaching against testing, using both, misusing neither.

Teaching and testing, caring and curing, this is the balance which you must seek in a physician.

EPILOGUE

Dehumanism /The Core of Our Discontent

"patients are people!"

Chapter Summary: Medicine has come a long way scientifically and technologically but it has wandered far off the beaten path so far as the human aspects of medical care are concerned. The spark of humanism burned out of the old GP's head and heart shortly after the Second World War and so much needs to be revived. How this will come about, when it will happen, and where the forces will be that will bring it about are not clear. I am attempting in this epilogue to point out the problem and hint at another book at another time where I hope to define it all a little further and point in some rational direction

---

Not long ago I hurriedly examined a nervous and pale little sixteen-year-old boy referred to me with abdominal pain. David was his name, but I didn't know that then. I had been asked by his pediatrician to examine his abdomen because of a suspicion of appendicitis. I found no evidence of any abdominal disease and recall making a mental note that the patient acted almost hysterical. I dismissed him and mother rather abruptly with a firm, reassuring but curt statement which amounted to, "Nothing is wrong, Mother, he's just nervous."

Two months later I went through the same ritual with this boy, still unable to pin anything down and still convinced he was a young neurotic. This time I admitted him to the hospital, ran off an abundance of examinations, all normal, and discharged him again.

David persisted. He showed up in my office a third time, about six months later, still complaining of vague abdominal pain. Somewhat perturbed, I lectured his mother in front of the patient. I explained that I was a surgeon, that I found no surgical problem with David, that he ought to be seen by some other kind of doctor. I suggested, rather subtly, a psychiatrist.

I shall never forget his mother. She looked down, anguished, turned to her son, and said, "Shall we tell him, David?" **In an instant I knew that whatever he revealed would not have been discovered by my laboratory or X-ray examinations**. I knew that I hadn't given him the time to relate, that I had failed this person by making him a nonperson.

In this case the revelation was that David was a heroin addict. But that's not the important thing. It could have been any one of a number of equally serious problems that will not surface until the patient is ready and confident enough to bring them forth.

"**Patients are people.**" You have to keep telling yourself that. It's so easy to forget in the course of a day's work. Medicine has become so uniform and standardized, specialized and organ-centered, that people are being forgotten. It's like the supermarket idea—plenty of quick service and efficient handling of orders—but it's all for nonpersons. They come in droves, pass blankly from one counter to another, are served with an automated smile, and they leave.

"Patients are people; diseases don't exist in things." You have to keep saying it twenty or thirty times a day. Each person is different. Each has his or her own bundle of troubles, collection of anxieties, and heaps of apprehensions. Some of them pretend to blot out their fears at first, and it's tempting to pretend with them. You have so little time for each one. It's simpler and quicker not to get involved. There are so many waiting to see you out there. Your secretary presses you on: "There's a gall bladder in room two." All that's needed is a quick appointment with the X-ray man, then schedule her for surgery. That's how the supermarket does it: five dollars for twelve cucumbers! Why can't the doctor do it this way?

Yes, why can't the doctor sell cucumbers? Why this insistence on a personal doctor-patient relationship? Apparently people want it that way. You hear the doctor described as cold, indifferent, mercenary and a host of other epithets all suggesting that he has lost sight of the real goal, the person he treats. These charges are not the product only of chronic malcontents, sensational journalists and authors of little consequence. The criticisms arise from sober sources. These critics point to various national polls and sociological studies pointing to one complaint of the public against the medical profession: **dehumanism**. It is the core of discontent, expressed in many ways but always meaning the same: **"The doctor doesn't know me as a person"; "I doubt that the doctor remembers who I am half the time"; "He's more interested in my appendix than my name."**

It would be a serious misconception to view these complaints as petty. The charges go deeper than the words used to express them. These people are not so insecure as to bemoan the loss of a chatty, friendly doctor. While such an arrangement may be attractive, patients do not consider it essential enough to worry about its loss. Criticism as a disinterested technician is rooted in an abiding belief that medicine can only be good when the person rather than his disease becomes the physician's focal point. Conversely, bad medicine is equated with depersonalized medicine and the majority of charges against the physician are corollaries of this equation.

But is this so? Imagine an advanced technological society in which the patient, highly sophisticated about disease processes, feeds his symptoms into a computer and receives diagnosis, prognosis and treatment printout cards. Impersonal? Yes, but wouldn't the disease respond to therapy just as well? The astronaut, his organs wired into highly sophisticated diagnostic sensors, whirls through space thousand of miles from his space physician and yet receives excellent though depersonalized medical care.

This raises the question about the nature of disease, its psychic components, and its consequences to the personality. We know what disease does to the personality. It does not exist in a vacuum and cannot be managed this way. The computer and the relay sensors will continue to improve our diagnostic and therapeutic skills. Technology is unlimited and will serve man's medical needs with increasing powers and with marvelous efficiency. But technology divides and analyzes to conquer. It will need to be offset by increasing personalism if we are to avoid an impossible distortion of human nature by some future head-on collision with the machine. Future man cannot permit the machine to invade his person and bring about "technological man," that electronic myth projected by too many social writers today.

Depersonalized medicine is bad medicine and there is already too much of it around. The psychosomatic nature of disease has been recognized in various masks since the Medicine Man first attempted to soothe and calm his patient with magic and prayer. Our failure today is a failure to recognize that only a personal, warm, and thoroughly concerned relationship with the patient can cure or control the entire disease process.

The cardiac patient requires a prolonged personal relationship with a sympathetic physician who follows the life-style of his patient and advises her, as circumstances dictate, as to the relationship between her cardiac condition and the life she's leading. Too casual a regimen could lead to cardiac failure and death; too strict, to cardiac neurosis, often more crippling than the disease itself. The line between the two is finely drawn. The physician learns only after a lengthy involvement with his cardiac patient just how much leeway he can give her, how responsible a patient she is, how stable, how neurotic, how tense. One executive can carry on a great deal of highly complicated business without stressing her heart, only to feel dangerously sustained stress in a competitive golf game. It is often far easier to diagnose the cardiac condition in the first place than to detect what specific activities stress this particular patient. Such information comes out of no computer and is subject to no known technology.

People grasp this principle of dealing with disease, which is at the root of their growing criticism about impersonalism and dehumanism in modern medical practice. They feel uncomfortable, for example, about the strange physician advising them when their own physician is on vacation or "off duty." They are hesitant about emergency surgery, until their own doctor sees them and okays it.

This isn't sentimentalism or a desire for bygone days. People just reason from their own professions or trades and realize that continuity, so essential a part of quality work for them, must be necessary also for the physician. They also know enough about disease to realize that it is affected by the lives they lead, their habits, their stresses, and so on.

Humanism is even more important in the management of psychosomatic and psychoneurotic disease. Here the total evaluation of the patient and his unique personality characteristics are inseparable from the symptoms he manifests. Diagnosis and treatment of these conditions is altogether impossible in some of our assembly-line clinics. A thorough analysis of the whole patient is the essence of good management. These illnesses are often illogical and non-scientific, and therefore cannot be programmed into a technological device with any anticipation of success. **Sometimes the most important part of therapy is the person of the physician rather than her drugs. Tragically, psychiatrists have now totally lost the idea of talk rather than drugs! The cost-controllers do not pay for talk; hence, no talk!**

Humanism is more than an attractive wrapping for unattractive science. It stems from the physician's attitude toward the patient, how she credits the worth of her patient as a person. Her approach to the patient will succeed to the degree to which she conceives of her patient as someone higher than the molecular level of chemical and biological law and higher than the psychological and behavioral level of hidden drives and distorted motives.

The public charges that medicine has become stark, drab and dehumanized. I believe this is a legitimate charge. But I also see an early awareness of the problem, a new consciousness permeating the medical profession, and this suggests that change for the better is just ahead. Whether spurred on by the demands of the public or responding to some innate decent voice, the medical profession has begun to take note of its own dehumanized system, and corrective measures are underway.

In the meantime, you must decide how "humanized" your physician really is. Does she treat you as an object, a thing needing repair, or as a fellow person in need of healing? Does she recognize your humanity as the purpose of her professional life or simply tolerate it as an inconvenient but necessary condition for the exercise of her technical skill, the fattening of her wallet or the gratification of her ego?

This human dimension in the doctor-patient relationship is something that you can sense if you look for it. If it's there, it means that your doctor values life and health—a necessary precondition of her value to you. If it's not there, not all of the technical competence or academic expertise in the world can take its place—**and you're in dangerous hands.**

How to choose a good doctor?

Look for a good person!